LOSING TIME

AIDS LESSONS IN LOVE AND LOSS

LUCIEN L. AGOSTA

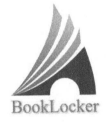

BookLocker

Saint Petersburg, Florida

ISBN: 978-1-64438-911-9

Published by BookLocker.com, Inc., St. Petersburg, Florida.

Author's Note: All people in this memoir are actual persons, though names have been changed for those who can no longer grant permission for their identities to be revealed.

Library of Congress Cataloging in Publication Data
Agosta, Lucien L.
LOSING TIME: AIDS LESSONS IN LOVE AND LOSS by Lucien L. Agosta
Biography & Autobiography/LGBT | Health & Fitness/Diseases/AIDS & HIV | Family & Relationship/Death, Grief, Bereavement
Library of Congress Control Number: 2019909022

Printed on acid-free paper.

BookLocker.com, Inc.
2019

TABLE OF CONTENTS

INTRODUCTION

I

Many gay men who survived the AIDS crisis of the 1980s and 90s still thumb a blister of grief and rage and guilt:

Grief over the senseless squander of hundreds of thousands of amiable, talented young men, our friends, our lovers.

Rage at Ronald Reagan, Senator Jesse Helms, and other politicians of their ilk in unholy alliance with Jerry Falwell and the indifferent religious hypocrites who averted their eyes and turned their backs on our suffering, avowing that our holocaust was an appropriate Biblical punishment meted out for gay sexual abominations. Reagan did not even mention the word AIDS until his friend Rock Hudson was stricken and then only after 53,000 Americans had already died of the disease, Americans he had pledged to serve and protect. And Falwell and his bunch so compassionately referred to people battling AIDS as WOGS (or Wrath of Gods).

Guilt that somehow we survived the plague by sheer dumb luck. "Survivor's guilt" they've termed it.

Why us, we ask? Why not Gordon, whose violin could scour the grime away from our lives while helming an orchestra as its first chair? Why not Carl, who earned an MFA from the Corcoran Gallery in printmaking a year before going blind from CMV (cytomegalovirus) retinitis and whose final gallery exhibition was held posthumously, as if to rub it in how much we had lost when he gave up the world he had so richly depicted? Why not Roger, whose idea of exalted living was a boozy night out at a South of Market gay grunge dive in San Francisco where he could be the piss-pig-cum-dump slut he prided himself on being? Or Declan, who soared a single season as lead in a ballet company before a fatal dose of PCP (pneumocystis carinii pneumonia) brought him low? Why not Connor, a broker at Charles Schwab who persuaded so many gay men into giving up their monthly paycheck sprees to establish long-term retirement investment plans, when, as it turned out, nothing long-term awaited them? Why not you, Dore?

So many fell out of history before they could make it. So many of us who have survived cannot get over it.

For a long time I avoided writing of my experiences during the AIDS crisis, still numbed by the repeated blows inflicted by the virus and needing a stay from a more intense engagement with it that writing of it would involve. Unprocessed grief always seeks a way out, though. The history of the AIDS era, which began nearly 40 years ago, has been largely outlined in works by Randy Shilts *(And the Band Played On)* and more recently by David France *(How to Survive a Plague)*. But dozens of my friends and acquaintances vanished unrecorded. For many survivors, still traumatized, closure escapes us: we live in a wide fracture. The thrust of memory of the Losing Time, its unimaginable magnitude, has gradually distilled for me with a gathering intensity that urges me to remember and record before memory blurs. Catastrophes like AIDS become meaningful or understandable only when humanized, when records of experience show how those catastrophes impacted specific human lives. Thus, though the general parameters of the AIDS crisis have been mapped, the particular human significances of that crisis still need to be told.

My experience centers in Sacramento, a city on the periphery of AIDS-epicenter San Francisco, an easy 80-mile drive regularly taken by scores of Sacramento gay men on weekends. Thus Sacramento bore in its gay populace the concussive blows from the infected Mecca just down the freeway. I moved in a milieu of mostly white, middle-class gay men, knowing few women or people of color who fought the virus in my time, though some were clients of the Sacramento AIDS Foundation where I volunteered with many tireless men and women, mostly gay, but some compassionate straight people as well. So I pen a parochial piece of AIDS history, a microcosm in the world of harm wrought by the virus. The novelist Garth Greenwell wrote in a recent article in <u>Out Magazine</u> that "we're at this really interesting moment of negotiating the narrative of the AIDS crisis for queer people in the 80s and 90s, and yet that story is only told about San Francisco and New York." This book answers Greenwell's desire for a part of the broader AIDS story to be told as well.

Coined in 1987, the powerful catchphrase "Silence=Death" indicated that a passivity of speech and action guaranteed the deaths of those battling AIDS, thereby threatening an entire beleaguered community. Over 658,000 people have died of AIDS in the United States alone since 1981, most of them gay men. Potent life-extending drugs have been developed and released as a direct result of the confrontational demands and anarchist tactics of Larry Kramer and others involved in the founding of ACT UP (AIDS Coalition to Unleash Power) and other activist groups, unwilling to be silent and passive any longer.

Today, when many people with HIV are living longer, indeed indefinitely, "Silence=Death" takes on an added significance: when the stories and the names of those lost to AIDS are forgotten, when silence cancels their memory, then they die the final death. Silenced irrevocably are their lives and the particular history of our times. Silence=Death indeed.

This book thus has a double, interrelated focus: First, and more broadly, it presents life as lived in Sacramento, CA during the AIDS crisis—the Losing Time of the title. As such it chronicles the lives of some of those doomed to lose time entirely during that awful epoch of the 1980s and 90s. Second, the book deals in some detail with the later life and too early death from AIDS of one man among the many remembered here—Dore Tanner (1949-1998)—who taught me in that dark era that love was more than the heterosexual illusion I had always believed it to be. Losing Time offers an honest, sometimes humorous, depiction of two gay men who blundered haplessly into a love neither of them was looking for and, subsequently, the fat grief that comes from so soon losing a lover so lately found and the determination it takes to find one's way again when one's compass points only south. The book's interweaving of particular loss with the many other casualties of that time presents the texture of life as Dore and I and so many other gay men we knew lived it during the Losing Time, which began nearly 40 years ago. The book's focus on personal experience provides the germ of a history already being generalized, its particulars fast being lost to memory.

I was no leader during that time. I offered no new ideas or strategies or tactics, never committed any acts of civil disobedience, never put myself on the line. I was a foot soldier, a mere functionary, a follower. A witness, though not, I am proud to say, an inactive one. A servant, I hope. Certainly no hero, though I strove together with valiant individuals in a common cause.

HIV has no cure yet, though its ravages today are held in abeyance for many in the United States, an uneasy lull in a slower carnage now occurring largely off stage. This leads to AIDS being viewed with a dangerous complacency by younger gay men and by society at large. A sobering 15,807 people died in the United States in 2016 of AIDS-related complications. Still. Many of us who survived are now striving, like me, to remember with a long-withheld acceptance the shock of the Losing Time before time itself overwhelms us. This account—improbable love story, memory vault, regenerative narrative—is an attempt to let go of that time at last without losing forever those no longer with us.

Other survivors of the Losing Time are now also empowered to give up their stories in whatever ways they can. The internet, social media, archival oral histories, podcasts, and self-publishing provide powerful modern outlets for relating the transformative narratives that give voice to our loss and restore us to history. Such deeply personal accounts provide the foundation of a history that must not be forgotten.

II

Dore Tanner: I address you directly in these pages. To reference you only in third person brings with it a distancing from you, an impersonal objectification I still do not feel, though you have been dead for over twenty years.

During your last weeks, you talked, with such extraordinary grace and courage, the life you were leaving. Early life and late you told out, the jumble of memory, that uncouth recorder that minds no order. Ever an accountant, after you had opened your life's ledger, you scanned the columns, canceled entries, shifted the figures, worked towards the final balance. And you got there. Your last night was mostly silence.

I am attempting in these pages what you did: I am telling my life with and without someone who can no longer speak for himself, with and without others who are now also mute. I am telling of life during the Age of AIDS: you stand forefront among the many lost with you with claims to be remembered as well.

I did not know you all that long, a scant two years total, though in the Age of AIDS, that was often considered a lengthy connection. Relationships had to be expedited in that fatal time, as ours was. By rights, I should have gotten over you long ago, settled things between us, resolved us. But I have come to know that some relationships end without resolution, end in a forced closure with lingering resonances and echoes that will not be stilled. In such relationships, no one else can ever occupy that unresolved place after it has been emptied, though life can be lived fully and richly even over that vacancy, and others can enter one's life to enrich it.

Now, as to this book: I am more interested in telling the truth than in reporting facts. Granted, facts are important, but one must always structure remembered events so as to locate the truth hidden within. What is importantly human can never be completely factual. As soon as the mind notices them, facts blur and transpose: events haze in interpretation, angle of vision, subjective filtering. All sleight of hand. These pages offer a necessary mix of memory and imagination and narrative sequencing. I have worded conversations to dramatize what I think you and I and others meant or intended to say. These pages are readings of moments re-visioned, told now in a language unavailable to me while those moments were occurring. I am telling the truth in the best way I know how to invent it.

III

Beside our bed you kept an old Chinese cabinet as a lamp stand. Its scuffed red-lacquer front bore bronze double-happiness pulls on four drawers, their interiors stained black. In them we piled a jumble of ticket stubs, love notes left on pillows, business cards, appointment reminders, airline flight itineraries, credit card slips, concert programs, receipts, party invitations, stock prospectuses, Valentines, paid bills, to-do lists, birthday cards, recipes, packets of photographic negatives, stray condom wrappers, too, too many obituaries and memorial programs—all the traces of our living together through the Losing Time.

You lived just long enough for us to fill the four drawers.

"There's a reason the drawers are lacquered black inside," you said. "They're black holes. Put something in that cabinet and it disappears. We'll never see it again. It's the cabinet of all lost things. It'll drag you in some day too!"

On the Sunday we sorted through your clothes, I asked your sister Bonnie for the cabinet. It has stood next to my writing desk for over twenty years. One day I took out the top drawer and overturned its contents onto the floor. Every item I pulled out of the pile prompted me to start. I have been writing you and the others echoed there ever since.

Now that I am concluding this memoir, I am starting to dream of you, of others now long dead. Freud's work on dreams was a crock. I think it is counter-productive to snatch dreams back from the morning dissolution they drift to. Dreams are the debris the mind is chucking out. The mind relaxes its stern daytime hold and goes wacko in the night. In dreaming, the mind tries to amuse itself when it has nothing else to do, having given up bossing the body around, its lumbering daytime playmate. Nevertheless, my recent dreams seem eerily apt.

Several nights ago, I dreamed we went to a fundraiser at some church. Pearlene, the maid who worked in my childhood home in Louisiana, was dicing red bell peppers for a jambalaya simmering in a sugar kettle over an open fire, a wooden stirring paddle laid over the black iron rim. You had something to do with all this. You held out to me a tray of small steaks, fat-veins raying across them like the fortune-lines in human hands. Around us, sitting expectantly on folding chairs, were many of the men I knew who went away with you into the darkness. Your chair had a ruby glass rosary coiled on its empty seat.

Last night, I dreamed you were sitting on a black leather sofa in a gray room. You sat alone in the albedo light of before-dawn, or dusk, or just before a rainstorm, your eyes lowered, your hands holding a book that for some reason I did not want you to read. You sat beside the red lacquer cabinet from our bedroom, its drawers all open and empty. I watched you for a long time, both of us apart and perfectly still.

I am finishing this memoir now. I am giving it up. To my astonishment, I have become Love's apostle Paul, yours the bolt that knocked me off my high horse. Like Paul, I now know Love to be real, the most potent of the three necessary virtues. Hope anchors second after Love. Faith—in progress towards universal human advancement, world order, genuine and inclusive human tolerance, or environmental balance--is the rabbit virtue, ever tensed to dart away, its white scut a butt-star racing into a twilit thicket.

I hope this particular account of loss during the AIDS era of universal gay grief will echo for those who come after us, to those who laugh again after the mourners have left. That era must not be forgotten by those who follow us.

Even if this love story in the Losing Time must molder in some dusty gay archive somewhere, time's hostage, I hope someone will stumble upon it at some time and know the wonder it was to love you, the catastrophe it was to lose you and all those many lost with you, the living possible even after that.

PART I: GIVING UP

Love was a freakish venture in the plague years, an aberrant gambit as AIDS busied itself with aborting intimacy and parting lovers. The horror of AIDS was that love and death both used the same body portals to do their work. Fear and love make odd fuck buddies. But so it was: against all odds, untrue to type, and nearing fifty, I fell in love for the first time while AIDS raged unchecked around me. And to beat it all, I fell in love with a man whose defenses against the virus were all but depleted when I met him. That loving was costly. I grew from it. In spite of what I am about to tell, I would go through it all again, for to love, I learned, is recompense enough in itself even when love cannot ultimately win or solve or change anything much.

So this is a love story in a dark time. I never imagined I would ever write one. In the first place, I did not believe in love. Also, I was lousy lover material. I did not want a partner or a lover. I elected early on to live alone all my life in a taut contentment. Oh, I wanted to have sex and all, but I wanted the men I had sex with to leave in the morning— at the latest. I even had a separate bedroom in my house reserved exclusively for sex: the "trick room," I called it. It was the first bedroom to the left, just past the foyer. Some late nights, my trick and I got no further into the house than this.

I came home from fourth grade one afternoon and announced to my mother that I never wanted to get married. She told me years later that she had been startled by this news, but she had tried not to make too much of it.

"You don't have to decide that right now when you're only nine years old," she laughed. "One day, when you're older, you might just fall in love, like Daddy and me, and change your mind."

What happened next startled her even more: "No!" I screamed and threw myself onto the floor. "No! I won't ever fall down in love. I <u>won't</u> get married. No one can make me."

My mother had had to pick me up and hold me in her arms to stop my sobbing.

This is a love story. This is how it began:

I taught in the English department at Kansas State University in Manhattan, Kansas for ten years (1977-1987), relatively safe from the viral holocaust then devastating large American cities and clear-cutting gay men like timber. I moved to Sacramento in my late thirties to take a job at California State University in 1987. When asked why I left Kansas, I would reply: "I slept with all the gay men in Manhattan, quarreled with their wives, and had to leave." Actually I dated only one married guy. Get this: he was a "manure diversion specialist" at a feedlot. No joke. "My job is bullshit," he used to say. He rode a horse all day: very D. H. Lawrence, an earthy cowboy fetish. His wife at first tolerated our little rodeo. She even insisted on going to the Horseshoe Grill for dinner with us on two occasions. Suddenly she turned: "Get that steer out of the corral," she told him, "or I'll get the hell out of Dodge. I'd rather you went back to riding the bush boys in the park." She failed to realize that I was no threat: I was job hunting and strategizing a move. Anyway, I did not believe in love, certainly not with a man so matrimonially encumbered. And so bow-legged.

When I arrived in Sacramento in fall 1987, the AIDS epidemic was at full calamity. I was HIV-negative, a consolation of the Kansas sequester. The plague tempered my erotic exuberance a bit at first, but I soon shed my Midwestern reticence and hurled myself out there. I felt like one of the Hebrew children who, after roaming around deserts where they did not belong, crossed over into the land of milk and honey—or at least scented lube and semen. I wanted to be a sex object. I wanted to be used. A lot. I was not looking for love. That chimera ate people.

After a childhood, adolescence, even young adulthood of faggot shame and sexual-orientation denial, I elected promiscuous hedonism as a life goal. No more for me the creeping around, masturbating in the shower to the hot but tame bare-chested men snipped from Sears catalog underwear pages, the thin paper soon waterlogging in the steam to reveal bra-stuffed women on the other side of the page. Coming to the sexual revolution late, I now meant to have promiscuous hedonism guide my practice. I had lost time to make up, an interrupted puberty to rejoin—the adolescent sex I had denied myself on boy scout campouts and sleep overs and all that! I had to run to catch up to the parade, even if it was now resembling more and more a funeral procession. I reasoned that were I afraid to live fully now in my fading youth, I too would become, though in a less devastating way, also a casualty of AIDS.

I lived in a one-bedroom apartment in midtown Sacramento that first year: gay central. I could not open my door to arrive or leave at night without doors all around me opening. Every trick I brought home seemed to know someone in the building. "Hey, how's it hanging?" my tricks would ask one or more of my gay neighbors peering out of a door at us. "Haven't seen you around for a while." Those introductions often got me sleeping with the neighbors as well.

By November 1987, the Catholic impulse had surfaced in me again: I affirmed a devout faith in my wondrous new gay life—but as anyone with a lick of sense understands—faith alone cannot grant salvation. I lacked good works, enraptured as I was by the three D's: disco, drink, and dick. Here I was discoing at the Masque of the Red Death, screaming and carrying on, throwing back booze and bedding whomever while so many were falling all around me for those same earlier behaviors they had not known enough yet to protect themselves from. I had watched the AIDS epidemic devastate from the security of semi-rural Kansas, had learned about safer sex practices in the nick of time, had used condoms for so long now that merely uncrinkling one from its packet was itself a penis-pumping turn-on.

I noticed an ad in a local gay rag, <u>The Patlar</u>, soliciting volunteers for the Sacramento AIDS Foundation's "buddy" or "Hand to Hand" program: clients with advanced HIV disease were matched with volunteers offering them emotional or practical support. I signed up to offer practical support—driving clients to doctor appointments, mowing an occasional lawn, grocery shopping—naively thinking thereby to evade taxing emotional involvements. I passed an initial interview, the central question being "Why do you want to volunteer to work with men dying of a disease that must frighten you as a gay man?" The interview team concentrated on my answer like ants on a honey drop. "It's the central concern of my community," I answered. "I'm reaping the rewards of belonging to that community: if I can help those facing a disease I am lucky to have avoided, I want to do that. I know that can be satisfying as well." Or words to that effect. I know how to use my tongue for a variety of functions, formal as well as louche. "Without those satisfactions, you won't go far in this work," said the chief interviewer. "The job you're volunteering for is tough. When can you train?"

The sessions during my training in early February 1988 were thorough and intense, occupying a Friday evening and all day Saturday and Sunday. I remember the first exercise from the Friday session: the "Giving Up Exercise," conducted by a man dying of AIDS, as he informed us before beginning. He did not need to announce this because he had what I called, strictly to myself, the "Dachau profile": sparse, straw-like hair of an indeterminate color; hollow, haunted eyes under a corrugated, feverish brow; a sallow complexion, sunken cheeks, and hunched shoulders; bones prominent everywhere. "I'm one of the people you've signed up to work with," he said. "You see what I've got and how I look. Get used to it quick. We need your help, not your pity. If you're just bringing here a bleeding heart, don't come back tomorrow. Go work with puppies at the SPCA."

He directed us to compile a list of the ten things most important to us, to write each of these items on a blank index card, and then to arrange the cards in ascending order, from least important to most. What was most important to me? I struggled with the list. I had just acquired a car, my first ever: that went down as number one, or least important. Next came the apartment I had rented with all the cheap furniture I had hurriedly bought for it. Third was the money I had stashed away in various retirement accounts. My job came next, followed by what I noted on the fifth card as "a generally optimistic attitude/overall happiness and contentment." I remember the wording: this gift was hard to phrase. On the sixth card I wrote "friends," on the seventh, "family." The eighth, ninth, and tenth cards were difficult to order, but they fell out as follows: health, mobility, and independence (8); my eyesight (9); my mind (10).

Others were struggling as much as I to compose and then order their cards. After everyone in the room—all fifteen of us—had written, crossed out, shuffled our cards into order, carped and complained, the narrative portion of the exercise began:

"For a week, you've had difficulty climbing stairs. Even the half-flight from the underground parking garage to your office cubicle on the first floor of your building leaves you winded and wheezing. You have to rest on the landing for a full five minutes to get to your second-floor apartment, and that's when you're not schlepping up a sack of groceries. You're doctor noodles around but finally diagnoses you with PCP pneumonia and refers you to an AIDS specialist. After completing three days in intensive care on oxygen to stabilize you, you're flat on your back in a quarantined hospital room for a week. Nurses come and go in your room, staggering around you like astronauts in moon-suits or like workers cleaning up a radioactive nuclear meltdown site. You have only partial-coverage health insurance and a five-thousand-dollar deductible. Give up two cards."

I flipped my car card into a wooden box on the floor in the middle of the circle. The savings card followed it.

"After being discharged from the hospital, you cannot go back to work for at least three more weeks. Somehow your born-again Republican boss finds out that not only are you gay, but you have AIDS. Your co-workers are afraid they'll catch it from you. Too weak to move from your sofa, the TV remote in your hand, you remember a joke your boss told you once: 'What do you call a faggot on skates?' 'Dunno,' you had said, grinning too hard. 'Rolaids.' You had laughed. Give up two more cards."

I threw my job card onto the pile. Reluctantly, I gave up the apartment card too.

"Your family in Utah sends you a pamphlet from the prophet informing you that AIDS is God's neat little extermination plan to tidy up gay abominations. Or, your family's evangelical pastor, told of your plight, takes it upon himself to tote up your celestial loss-assessment balance sheet for you in figures fire-and-brimstone Revival red. Or, the Vatican announces in the world's newspapers that you are 'intrinsically disordered.' Your family clips the account and sends it to you with a yellow sticky attached, advising you that you blew it in this world and you better as hell reckon with the one to come by making a complete confession to a pedophile priest as soon as possible. Oh yes, and they add that they cannot come to visit you because they are afraid they will catch your AIDS. Give up two more cards."

I threw away the family card. The one with "generally optimistic attitude" followed it into the discard box.

"While running a bath, you notice a purple blotch just above your right ankle. It looks like this." The conductor of the exercise rolled back the sock over his right ankle to reveal an irregular raised blotch of bluish purple. "You dismiss it as a bruise: you stumbled over the vacuum cleaner or something. In the tub, however, you notice another behind your left knee, another on the inside of your right thigh, just below the permanently enlarged lymph node big and hard as a walnut in your groin area. Within weeks you develop Kaposi's sarcoma lesions on your nose, forehead, and cheeks along with a white bloom of thrush at one corner of your mouth. You're embarrassed to go out in public. You call your best friend. You tell him you're thinking of killing yourself. 'Oh don't do that!' he cries: 'Let's go shopping at Macy's when you look better. I'll call you.' He never does. Give up two more cards."

"Jesus!" I said to myself. The "friends" card went. The "mobility and independence" card followed. The cards in the box splayed to the side under a gathering weight.

"You wake up in the middle of the night. At least you think it's the middle of the night. Your vision is blurred by CMV retinitis. You think you're in the lobby of the Hyatt. You see people coming and going, a glass elevator whizzing up a wall in the atrium. A lady with blue hair walks towards you, carrying a vinyl suitcase red as a Valentine. 'What are you doing here in sweats?' she demands. You suspect she is not real: she jitters in and out of focus like an image on a television with rabbit ears near an airport. You know somehow that you are in your bed, but all the same you cannot get out of the Hyatt. You manage to dial 911. The paramedics bust open your front door chain-lock to get in. You think they are firemen in the Hyatt lobby. You panic and try to run for the exits. They have to restrain you. Your neighbors peek through the cracked-open doors of their apartments to watch you being rolled to an ambulance strapped to a gurney and raving. Give up your last two cards."

I lifted my left haunch and tucked the last two cards under it, the eyesight and the mind cards.

"You have to give them up," gruffed a top-heavy lesbian assisting with the training. She reached for them, but I whipped them out and held them behind my back.

"You too," she ordered the guy sitting to my right. He was holding onto one last card. It said "Lover" on it. I thought to myself, "Oh give up the card, stupid. Your 'lover' skedaddled the moment he first heard your bigot boss fired you." The lesbian pulled the lover card from his resisting fingers and tossed it on the pile.

"And that," concluded the implacable voice, "is the fate, give or take a dozen other variant disasters, of the people you are volunteering to work with."

The next morning, assembled early for coffee and gluey Danish for day two of the training, only eleven of the original fifteen of us sat down in the circle.

This is the story of one man who never believed in love, who disdained it as a sentimental heterosexual fiction evolved to keep a man and a woman together just long enough to raise their kids. That man, without warning, slammed into the solid thing he long thought void. That man at last gave up enough of his dented egoism to learn to love, to know how brave lovers have to be, how arduous it is to love well, more exhilarating and painful than he had ever imagined.

This is the story of another man in the process of losing time altogether, of giving up everything on this earth, but who, in spite of all that, had the grace and courage to accept and extend love for the first time ever on his way out.

This is the story of two men, buffeted by AIDS, but each playing a fast, full hand, indeed a whole deck, gambling for everything with their cards fanned in a flush. They won. This is the story of two men giving up in a Losing Time.

PART II: SETTLING FOR

EVERYTHING

THE WRECK ROOM

It had been a hell of a Friday. I had spent the better part of it with Sean, a person—or what was left of one—whom I had met only the week before. The AIDS Foundation had called to ask if I could sit with Sean once a week on a day when no home healthcare sitter could be provided for him, usually Friday afternoons. Sean had contracted PML (progressive multifocal leukoencephalopathy), a devastating AIDS-related neurological degeneration that had descended on him irreversibly during the course of several weeks. The first sign of trouble: a full coffee cup had slipped out of his hand as he lifted it at work. Then came dizziness so disorienting he could no longer stand up. Then he could no longer speak. Next came blindness. Then the tremors started, followed by frequent convulsions and seizures. By the time I met him, he was semi-comatose, strapped down at his home in a hospital bed. When I raised the head of his bed to feed him, he opened his mouth wide and whimpered like a hatchling. His tongue was blistered with oozing, uncontrollable herpetic stomatitis. He had to have his waste expressed by a visiting LPN every other day with a rubberized speculum.

"Sean'll be a short assignment," the case manager at the Foundation told me on that first call. "Prepare yourself: it's not pretty."

Directly from Sean, I went to dinner with Mary T. and Robert, friends of mine of long standing. They knew where I had been.

"We'll start with champagne!" Mary T. screamed as she swung the door open. "You need it!" Robert burped a cork in the kitchen.

We dined alone, the three of us. We talked books. They did not like any of the edgy operas in the San Francisco season this year.

"Who can listen to yet another *Carmen*," I asked. "And please: enough *Boheme* with its doomed and petty lovers! How about a little Glass or Adams? A new commission from Jake Hegge?"

"We're talking opera here," snapped Robert. "If I want to hear squeaks and snorts, I'll take a walk downtown among the homeless on the K Street Mall. There it's free."

"I like a little adventure in the opera house, as in the bedroom," I protested.

"We can, I hope, agree about Boito's *Mefistofele*?" Robert asked. "That production almost made me a Christian again."

"It certainly does not sentimentalize love," I said. "Mefistofele prides himself on never having loved, and Margherita would have done a hell of a lot better had she never loved either. Faust remains unredeemed by romantic love, only by a desire to benefit mankind."

"Speaking of love, how is Eric?" Mary T. asked.

"He dumped me a couple of weeks ago," I laughed. "He called up on a Monday evening and said, 'Lu, we need to talk.'"

"He dumped you on the <u>phone</u>?" screamed Mary T.

"'So, talk!' I told him. Then there was this long pause. 'Eric,' I said, to fill the silence, 'if you called to dump me, certainly you rehearsed what you wanted to say?'

'Don't put it that way,' he said.

'Okay,' I said. 'Let me help you out: Lu, I like you as a friend. We've had some good times together, but I'm just not ready for a relationship. You're a great guy and all....' How's that Eric? How am I doing?"

Another long silence.

"'Okay,' he said at last. 'I guess that's what I wanted to say.'"

"Now that wasn't so hard, was it? It's alright, Eric. We had a good time. The sex was terrific. I'll miss that."

Mary T. and Robert eyed each other.

"Oh, it wasn't the last scene in *Traviata*," I laughed. "I'll have a harder time saying goodbye to you two tonight."

I left at about 10:30, exiting the warm house into a tule fog so sticky that I could not clear it from the windshield. I needed a transfusion, a replenishment in the blood of that gay tonic leached out by a workweek fitted into the straight world. All gay people are uneasy tourists in that flat land, no matter how out we are. In the straight country, gay people have worker visas, emigrant passports. Some of us are undocumented aliens.

The first "AIDS benefit" was held in a gay bar as early as 1982, and gay bars have been centers of activism and community structuring when homophobia denied us any other viable places to come together to share our lives. The Sacramento AIDS Foundation had its origins in a mid-town gay bar. Thus, the gay bar for us during the Losing Time and before was embassy, home territory in a foreign country, a safe space. At least it was after Stonewall in 1969.

So, I was not ready to go home just yet. My house would be cold and silent, my bedroom bone-tinted in the dim light reflected from the gold-lacquered Chinese screen covering the far wall. Eric would not be there, nor would anyone else.

Eric and I had dated for over four months. The sex was randy, always a tussle amid tangled sheets, all systems go! Eric had spiked hair, bleached platinum; eyes one shade lighter than amber, almost orange; a body gym-toned but too narrow in the shoulders. His skin was the smooth color of the "flesh" crayon that used to be included in the big, politically incorrect Crayola box. He was nine years younger than me.

When I fucked him, which he preferred, he frowned, his eyes locked on mine, his mouth fallen open as if to protest. Sometimes he closed his eyes and turned his head on the pillow and moaned. Then I thrust harder. When he topped me, I positioned him so we could see ourselves in the mirrors on the closet doors. All that was over, and it was time.

Though I liked Eric, I liked being unattached better. I liked the electric tremor arcing through the air I moved in when unmoored. Every man I met outlined a new adventure. The gay world radiates potential, a hovering accessibility. Interest goes flaccid with habit. A perverse pleasure exists in accumulation. "I know him intimately-- but not well": I could say this of any number of men.

So, that November Friday night just before Thanksgiving, I was out to review the troops, to finger the goods, to call roll. I was there to grab ass and write down names. I was Crusoe looking for Friday. Huck seeking Jim. I wanted to hear again the song of my blood surge, align that song with a throbbing gay pulse, especially after my grim vigil with Sean all afternoon.

The Wreck Room was the darkest, dirtiest, sleaziest gay bar in Sacramento, and hands down, my favorite. I loved the name of the place, but what could it mean? Was it named for the human wrecks drifting to rest there each night, survivors of their lives' crashes—bitter divorces, estranged children, lost jobs, all for being gay? Was it named for literal automobile wrecks, sudden smashups shot out of the blind spot, their violence and noise at once appalling and perversely erotic? Was it named for the striking of lust out of the bar's darkness, or the chance collisions that I have been told can result in a deeper connection, spuming like a fantastic lotus out of the mud? Was it named in wry allusion to the Department of Motor Vehicles building looming directly across the street from it? Beats me.

The Wreck Room glowered like a dark, angry planet next to the Je T'Aime Shoppe, a long, narrow chamber to be avoided by the squeamish, a paradise of lewd titillation, a lubricious wonderland.

I loved to take inventory in the Je T'Aime Shoppe. Anal beads, sized from pearls to ping-pong balls, hung above a glass cabinet filled with squeeze devices for tit play arranged according to torture level, from flexible rubber snake-bite suction cups to serrated-metal clamps, toothed like alligators. Every conceivable kind of dildo shared this cabinet: some, marketed with names like "Thunder Dong" and "Goliath," exceeded all possible human dimensions to make those into fisting and even the most insatiable size-queens gasp.

There was more: black leather whips, prods, and paddles; chrome harnesses, handcuffs, cock rings, razors— a fetishist's shelf of bliss. Blow-up do-me dolls, mouths agape, were tethered high on one wall like perverse angels. Ranked beneath were butt plugs, penis enlarger pumps, vibrators, bottles of non-prescription potency pills, and enema equipment. And in a small side room, like a library, stood the porn videos, their titles little erotic grenades: *Sleeping Booty. Cockpit: Everybody's Going Down. Young Dick-Tator. I Dream of Weenie. School of Hard Cocks.* The twisted poetry of perversion.

The very existence of the Je T'Aime Shoppe suggested to me the real truth: "Love" is little more than a genteel cover-up for the promiscuous animal lust that goads us all. Let's call it what it is. And enjoy it. Lots of it.

I cruised the video room: Not much to work with tonight. I have picked up men in the Je T'Aime Shoppe: the light is right; the wares blunt and honest. You can often tell what a man is into by what he is buying. Placement is everything. Two naked bodies in my dim front bedroom plying tits and squeezing a tube of lube: Now that's what I called "Love"!

One entered the Wreck Room next door through wide straps of black leather, like the strip curtain on a meat freezer. The front door opened into a narrow room with the bar defining the right wall. Scattered tall tables in the middle passage allowed one to rest elbows and drinks while watching the flow through the room. Off a short corridor at the back, two johns radiated uremia and red light. Women were unwelcome here, so the johns, though marked for gender, were indiscriminately available.

A pool room paralleled the bar room. The back part of this pool room offered a dark seating area where desire was brokered, negotiations proceeded (top? bottom? fisting? tit-play? spanking? fetishes? my place? yours?)—

lust's busy salon. This room ended with two pool tables frozen like gigantic cockroaches caught in the beams of a bright spotlight. Racks of gay publications fluttered one back into the bar room, where one could round again the cruise circle or short-circuit out the front door.

Oh no, not just yet!

I ordered a Bud Lite and made the obligatory roundabout. Life quickened. Would I be prey or hunter tonight? Top? Bottom? Greek? French? Bilingual? The blood-lust exhilaration of fluent identity, of shifting roles, of perverse possibility—that unique sexual gift available to the gay man!

I lighted at a tall table where two friends of mine were standing with drinks. It is good not to appear lonely and pathetic in a gay bar, but when talking to a couple, it is important to position oneself in such a way as not to seem connected to either party.

Richard propped his jaw up with one hand: "So over this," he sighed. "Hoped for magic tonight; got tragic instead. As usual."

Dale pointed to a fat man anchored at the entrance to the johns. He had limped into the johns after me several times before and peered over the urinal divider.

"Roly-poly at his usual post," Richard said. "Old tea-room queen."

"Parked in your space?" I laughed. Richard regularly cased out the johns too.

"It's okay," he yawned. "Daddy's not in there yet 'cause the bitches ain't in heat till later."

Dale started talking about his kids. His son had just smashed up his new truck, given him as a high school graduation gift. He had leaned over to change a CD, had clipped a mailbox, sideswiped two parked cars, veered into a ditch. The kid was in a neck brace. And his daughter, Dale added, did not want him at her high school pep rally to see her crowned a homecoming princess: "They all know you're gay, Dad. They'll make fag calls."

"And to think I shelled out a hundred bucks for a tin and glass tiara no self-respecting drag queen would muss up her wig with," he lamented.

"Well, you're the one who went off and got married," said Richard. "Pussy! What were you thinking?"

Dale sighed: "Everyone conspired to make me think I was in love. You hope marriage is a way out of the gay thing."

Etiquette in gay bars permits gay men to converse with only an occasional glance at the person one is talking with. Gay men are at their bars to look at other men. It is required. In the straight world, one's gay gaze is necessarily covert and always guarded. In gay bars, the gaze is unfettered, wanders at will. Every experienced gay man understands the language of the look. A gay man in a gay bar frequently conducts two conversations at once, speaking with the person in front of him and at the same time signaling with someone else across the room through an ocular eloquence early acquired.

Gay bars offer a revelatory space where the truth of oneself is not in doubt. Presence in a gay bar is a heralding of being, an existential declaration. At least it was in my generation. Every gay man in the straight world moves through a matrix of duality. We work and live in the straight world, but we are really not of it. We are fitted by life with bifocal lenses. We are benign schizophrenics, double agents. We walk the straight world as resident aliens with green cards. We guard our gaze. We look for signs. We sense, through nuance, others like ourselves, passing.

Being in gay space fosters the refreshment of a unified field. For a change, we are what we see. But gay bars can be painfully cruel places as well. When gay vision is unified and freed, it often plays over surfaces. The old, the fat, the ugly—beware: gay gaze can be withering.

I once persuaded a married, bisexual friend of mine to have a drink with me in a gay bar. He was hesitant. "I'm too fat," Barry protested. "And I'm wearing this hideous yellow shirt my wife gave me for my birthday."

"We'll just sit quietly at the end of the bar and have a nice chat over a cocktail," I coaxed. "No one will be there on a Wednesday night."

Just through the front door of the bar we encountered a team of young gay men in baseball jerseys celebrating a league win. They parted to let us pass.

"The school bus has arrived," one of them snickered, gesturing at my friend.

Gay men make impossible demands of human flesh. We have a difficult time forgiving it for its perfidy: it <u>will</u> age (if one is lucky in the Losing Time); it <u>will</u> sag over the years. And gay men unaccountably forget, especially in the arrogance of youth, that all human bodies that way tend, in spite of the gym time. I have heard young gay men protest that when they reach forty, they would rather die than be found in gay bars, leering like trolls. Many will be in gay bars at fifty, at sixty, even well beyond this. They will move to Palm Springs, or choose old-man bars—"wrinkle rooms" or "museums"—the lucky ones will, the ones who make it through the plague.

I did not see you enter the bar. The Greek gods were incredulous at how strange it is to be human: "Foolish mortals," went their awed refrain, "you cannot see your fate even when it is upon you!" We are not cognizant, even in living them, of which moments will vanish, which will be fixed forever.

I caught you out of the corner of my eye. Our gazes locked. You had the look of one who had been blonde in your youth: adulthood, with its weight of jobs and houses and sex and taxes, darkens hair. Your summer tan was waning. Your eyes, unwavering on me without either aggression or hunger, were a spectral blue in the black-lighted dimness of the bar. I later knew them to be the color of shallow water on a silver day when the sun is chrome through cloud haze. Eloquent and legible eyes, they often revealed what you declined to speak. Your nose was long from bridge to narrow nostrils, a benign, masculine passage. A broad mouth based it, a full bottom lip bolstering a thin upper one—generosity tempering reserve.

I knew your type: you were a golden boy—but you seemed not to know it. Some repressive force, I surmised, had dimmed the usual glimmer around those aureate beings among whom you numbered. Conscious of their fortunate looks and of the admiration they prompt, golden boys glide through gay life. They never know a closed door. Though you had clear claim to it, you seemed never to have assumed their incandescence. Your gold seemed shadowed. Perhaps you came into this exaltation without being aware of your beauty?

Golden boys are incarnations of Teutonic gods: whatever ancient, atavistic sense of inferiority invests the southern Latin centers in me as well. Small, dark, hairy, at some deep level I have bought into the Wagnerian myth, Alberich to your Siegfried. A loose ease, a masculine gentleness invested you. You gazed at me in that bar from a composed center.

Gay gaze often lingers but may mean little: indifferent curiosity or mere sightseeing; a trial signal beamed to determine another's interest level; an early attraction withdrawn once a closer inspection reveals a fatal flaw, as minor as one's choice of drink or an unbecoming haircut, as major, for me, as drunkenness or effeminacy or bad teeth. I returned your gaze. You walked past me and through the passage into the pool room.

Now on alert, I chatted with my friends, the verbal flow unchecked. And then you passed again, eyes full on me.

"Somebody's getting heavy cruised!" said Richard. "When someone looks at you that hard, he either wants to eat you or fuck you. It's nature's way."

"Maybe you'll get lucky and he'll do both," said Dale.

You passed through the doorway into the pool room again and stopped just inside.

"You are dismissed," said Dale, fluttering his fingers to usher me away. "Take precise notes and let me type them up."

You were alone, waiting, half in, half out of a dark sexual vestibule. I turned from my friends without a further word, another prerogative sanctioned by unconnected gay men conversing in our bars, and walked toward where you were waiting. My first step toward you brought you to me.

Lu.

Dory.

Like the little flat-bottomed boat?

Flat-bottomed?

Isn't a dory a boat?

You're the first to make that connection.

Do you live in Sacramento, Dory?

I do. And you?

In College Greens.

We're neighbors! I live in Glen Brook.

Practically next door. I was at dinner with friends tonight. It ended before I was ready to go home.

I was at a Bears game-night with my friend Tim. (Bears are burly, hirsute, generally older gay men. You were no bear!)

Hunting? Hibernating? Playing Goldilocks?

Oh, I'm not into Bears. I left early.

So what do you do?

I work for the State. I feed at the trough, like every other man here.

Like me.

Which department?

I teach English at Cal State.

I work for the Bureau of State Audits.

Pardon the obvious question, but are you an auditor?

I'm a fraud investigator.

I've got nothing to hide.

Everyone does.

Even you?

I take the fifth. Want to frisk me?

Here?

Well, I own a house....

You were looking for someone to share this one night with, to come with you into your silent house and stir the air with laughter and low murmurs. You wanted a one-night adventure, your usual habit. Mine too. But I turned uncustomarily shy. Intimidated, unusual for me. And it was late. Hell, I am not sure why I did not go home with you there and then. I suspect that if I had gone home with you that first night, I would have disappeared into the pattern, been labeled "trick" and dismissed. I liked that game too, in so many ways so satisfying, sex so uncomplicated. I have discarded business cards as soon as the door closed behind men I have just fucked.

I left you in the Wreck Room that Friday night in the certainty that love was a heterosexual fever dream, a tall tale, a hoax. Fickle, fascinated with sex, eschewing human complexity and claims, I sought pleasure, always willing to give it to get it. But in the Wreck Room that night, I had a collision with what I would come to recognize as the real, though I would not realize the impact of that crackup for some time. My lightsome blood would thicken on later learning what coiled in yours, had insinuated itself into your very DNA like the poison sap from the apple eaten in Eden. The knowledge of love and death was seeded in me during those minutes with you in the Wreck Room that night. I was to learn in you the resonantly human at last, its text of sorrow and joy. Human fullness would in time be love-taught.

A SEA CHANGE

Sunday evenings are melancholy expanses, especially in winter after sunset spreads a blue smudge over a bleached western horizon. The mind flattens forward into the coming workweek after its float in untethered weekend time. A phone ringing in a darkening room rouses one from late Sunday lethargy.

How to open? Just dial and let instinct take over. Rehearsed gambits never work. The other person cannot follow a script he has never read.

"Dory? This is Lu. We met Friday night?"

"I was this very minute walking across the room to call you."

"You weren't really, but what a happy thing to say."

"I was really."

We made a date for Thursday, a week after Thanksgiving. On that day, I walked home from teaching with a hammering headache along a gray river in a bitter drizzle. My house was cold and dark. A hot shower, I thought, would make me feel more like meeting you.

A half hour before I was to leave to meet you at the café, you phoned to ask if I would mind picking you up. Car trouble. I considered this a sly preamble. On several occasions in my long dating career, I had picked men up at their front doors who answered the knock draped in towels, seemingly fresh from the shower, "running late." They had wanted sex before sustenance. The wares were on display. I was always gallant: "Can I have a drink first?"

You answered the doorbell—fully dressed, apologizing for putting me out. You did not invite me in.

We drove to midtown down streets wet and slick as seal backs, taillights Technicolor-red as a Hawaii sunset in an Elvis movie. Café Bernardo glowed an Old Master brown-gold, its walls hung in seascapes by a local artist deficient in both inspiration and talent: Lighthouses leaked light into fog banks, that sort of thing.

We ordered at the back counter, polenta and ratatouille, a glass of red wine for me; beef stroganoff on caraway-buttered noodles for you.

"Are you vegetarian?" you asked, your brow furrowed. "Or, God forbid, vegan?"

"What would Oktoberfest be without bratwurst? Or Thanksgiving without turkey? Sex without swallowing the sausage? No, I'm not vegetarian."

"That's a relief," you said, "and enticingly put."

We took a table close to the front door. We had been given a playing card stuck in a metal coil to stand on the table so the server would know where to bring our food—the three of hearts.

"Lucky number," I said.

"Why lucky?"

"It's a sacred number. And the hearts...."

"Are you religious?" you asked.

"I'm religious, not spiritual," I said.

"Don't you mean that the other way around?" you asked, eyebrows raised.

"No. I'm a cradle Catholic."

"Practicing?"

"Perfected."

The server brought our food: "Dore! Haven't seen you in ever so long!"

You looked up, surprised. "Bert? Are you working here now?"

"Yeah, I had to take this second job after my health insurance dropped me. Fortunately they covered that bitch of a meningitis episode that put me in the hospital a couple of months back. Cryptococcal. The bad kind. Those fungal buggers mobbed my brain stem with Uzis and hijacked it."

"I hadn't heard."

"I had had this wracking headache all day. By evening after work, it felt like my skull was thin as a cracked eggshell and I had trouble moving my neck. I had never had such pain. Fortunately Tom called me that evening and found me gibbering nonsense. He thought I was trying to speak Russian, of which I know not one word. He came right over and took me to the emergency room. There, apparently, I put on quite a show: out of my mind and shouting before they rushed me away from the little Mexican abuelas clutching their grandchildren away from me. I don't remember any of this, not even the seizures that followed. When the insurance company discovered the meningitis was AIDS-related, they dropped me, the bastards."

"Is that legal?" I asked. "Can an insurance company do that?"

"It is, and they can. I consulted a lawyer about it, and after poring over my contract and drilling the insurance company, she concluded that it was both chickenshit AND legal. That amounted to a $500 consulting fee."

Bert looked at Dore: "You don't have anything to worry about on this score. The State takes good care of their own, like any good mother, right? But hey," he continued, "this could have been a lot worse: at least my boss at the tech firm hasn't made any move to fire me yet, probably because he's gay and thinks I got screwed. He can't get the insurance reinstated, though. Now I've got a crapload of doctor bills and the attorney fee, so here I am slinging hash. You're leaving me a generous tip, right?"

The front door shushed open and closed as we ate, the chill caustic with car exhaust. My headache, the hammer wrenched away from it by three aspirins, gave a few half-assed knocks but failed to hit the nail. No meningitis there.

"Okay," I said. "You first. Who the hell are you?"

You were working two-thirds time as a fraud investigator for the California Bureau of State Audits, part sleuth, part report-writer. You had retired in your mid-forties when the Auditor General's Office had been disbanded after the passage of a cockeyed voter proposition. Since a state cannot run without an auditing agency, the Bureau of State Audits was soon constituted to replace the old agency, and you, bored silly in a too-early retirement, agreed to return part time as a "permanent intermittent CPA." You delighted in the absurdity of your classification.

Bureau investigations of fraud in state agencies were ruthless and thorough. Over a long career, you had become a master at scenting out the dodges and cover-ups of those less proficient at cheating than you were at tracking it.

You were a Libra. You were a year and three months younger than me. You could not remember ever having dated an older man. "For several months of each year, you will be two years older than me and therefore a cougar," you said.

"Do you plan to make much of that fact?"

"Oh, I promise to," you said. "Your turn."

"Do you prefer to interview me, or may I give a deposition?"

"Either way, you're under oath."

I described the four classes I taught on Tuesdays and Thursdays.

"You work only two days a week?"

"Okay," I said, "here's the deal: I teach two days a week. On the other days I prepare for classes, respond to piles of student papers, do research and write, and attend committee meetings. There's no need for your Bureau to launch an investigation."

"I'm placing your case in the inactive file," you said.

I told you about having taught for ten years at Kansas State before coming to California.

"I'll bet you were happy to have escaped Kansas," you said.

I let it go. "I left because I wanted to live in a larger gay community. But I liked my job there, and besides, being tucked away in Kansas for most of the 80s insulated me from AIDS. I know if I'd been in California during those years, I'd probably be dead by now."

"I have it."

I looked down.

"I've lived with the virus for a long time," you added.

I sat sideways to the table, my eyes roving the room. Something formless and troubling was squatting on the table between us: I did not want to look at it.

I took you home, declined to come in.

"I can't," I said when you asked me out for Saturday night. I was working that weekend in Oakland, scoring papers for a national educational testing service. I would not be back until late Sunday.

The deliberations about that first date ended in a draw. You were smart and kind and stable. I liked you. You were my physical ideal: the Teutonic knight. You moved like a slender swimmer through water. Your eyes were the pale shallow of ocean surge above sand. Your large sexy hand curled on the table like a conch shell. The dark, hairy, short Italian seeks the resplendent Austrian, the golden-haired conqueror on Sicily's beaches.

That was all in one pan of the scale.

In the other pan: HIV. That pan weighted heavy.

When I returned from work on Sunday, you had left a message on my machine: "Let me reciprocate dinner. Tuesday evening at my house, after your classes?"

"I'm so glad," you said when, after hesitating, I called to accept. "Do you like seafood?"

"All kinds," I answered.

"Oysters?"

Aphrodisiac.

You had a fire crackling in the living room off the entry. The granite of the fireplace surround glimmered like a black opal. The lights were dim.

I asked for a martini. You did not have gin, vermouth, olives, martini glasses, or a shaker. (You had them the next time I came over. You learned to love that clean, crisp cocktail too.)

You were looking through cookbooks, casting about for an entrée to serve to your fifteen colleagues at a departmental Christmas party you were hosting the following Saturday evening.

"This one," I said. "Definitely this one." I pointed to the recipe for chicken in champagne sauce from the *San Francisco a la Carte* cookbook.

"You do know what this means? Fate is in charge here, not coincidence. This is one of my favorite recipes."

"If fate ruled," I said, "we'd be clinking stemmed glasses over second martinis."

Your face fell.

Later, after dinner, when I stood to leave, I gave you a brisk hug. You ran your fingers lightly over my forearm. "Do you really have to go? You don't teach tomorrow."

"It's been a busy, long day," I said.

I am certain that I had slept with men infected with HIV before. In fact, I considered every man I tricked with in California as harboring the virus. I always took precautions. Somehow <u>knowing</u> you were infected changed everything.

"Come for dinner Saturday night. You'll like the people I work with."

"What to do? What to do?" I asked myself for several days. On Friday morning before reporting at Sean's, I went to the AIDS Foundation to file a depressing update on him. His case manager told me what I already knew: safer-sex practices work. Serodiscordant couples can have thrilling sex. (She called such couples "electric": the infected partner positive, the other negative for the virus.) Both partners can stay healthy. She gave me a sack of condoms, some lube. "Make love well," she said.

All that Friday afternoon sitting with Sean, now clearly dying, his tremors stilled though with occasional seismic episodes, I thought that dating needs to be easier than this. Here was Sean himself, emblem of what AIDS could do—to you, to me.

But there was something else as well, something I could barely admit to myself, never to the caseworker: I fought against an instinctive inclination to stigmatize those infected with HIV, to question their moral worth. I disguised a tendency, of which I was ashamed, to assign those positive with HIV to some kind of viral underclass, to judge them as tainted through their own doing. My work at the AIDS Foundation thus involved a guilt-laden brew of compassion, judgment, and revulsion. Fear too. Even more centrally, it involved a deep relief on being myself free of the virus, some measure of distaste for those I wanted to serve, guilt for these feelings that would force themselves upward in a psyche trying hard to dispel them, a psyche infected by the prejudices and judgments of the larger culture that shaped it. To this toxic brew was also, undoubtedly, a residual internalized homophobia and self-hatred for being gay.

What surprises me in retrospect is that I did not add to this awful mix any concern about the burden that would fall to me were you to get sick—really sick—if we were to enter into any kind of a relationship. I could walk away from Sean after an afternoon—with enormous relief—as I had been able to do with others I had been assigned to help through the AIDS Foundation. Somehow I did not think much about a long stretch of being primary caregiver and extending those often loathsome tendernesses to someone full time. Perhaps I failed to factor this possibility into my deliberations because on the horizon were promising new drugs that were extending life, even for those toeing the grave's abyss. You were taking them. In spite of this promise of new, life-extending meds, I was still attending a memorial service at least once, occasionally twice or more, every week or so.

I projected that every time we had sex, I would worry about getting infected. And was not sex what this was all about? Had I not decided early on that "love" was an ephemeral coalescence of infatuation, an envious annexation in another of what one lacked in oneself, lust, of course—all in just the right fickle suspension to produce a heated intensity? For the time being. So, "love" for me was delicious but not very filling, a soufflé: a combination of ingredients and flavors, the right timing and temperature, a hunger in that moment for the airy confection. But "love," like a souffle, could never last. The first forkful deflates it. Except for tasting tongue and sucking dick, I never cared much for "French" comestibles.

What to do? What to do?

On Saturday morning, Phyllis, my close friend from Kansas days, told me not to get involved. "Stop this before it gets started," she counseled. "Can't you find someone to fuck who's not lethal?"

That evening I thought I would not go to your party. I decided—definitively--that it would be better if I just let all this go.

I arrived at your house around 9:00. Everyone was still eating. I watched you so intently throughout the evening that I hardly interacted with anyone else. They were all straight anyway. You sat at the far end of your oval table so as to get to the kitchen easily. Sidelined, you were central. Guests sought you out. That was important to me: I always wanted to be with someone popular, someone of whom others approved.

Office stories revolved around you. Someone told how you once booked a session with a state worker you were investigating on a tip that she was conducting private sexual massages for pay while she was on the clock. You helped her set up her table and taped her as she told you exactly what she would do for you for $100. She had pleaded with you when you told her she was busted, one of those you felt sorry for once they were nabbed. In another of these sad dramas, you fingered a man in the insurance commission who tried to steal three office computers and the office dolly he had trundled them out with.

"Do you have to go? Stay," you said when I rose to leave with the rest of your guests.

I knew that you were growing impatient. You had rightly surmised that I was so spooked by the virus that I would try to convert our connection into some sort of platonic frustration.

"Don't give up yet," your friend Tim counseled. "If you're interested, give him more time."

Sunday morning I mulled you over, sipping strong coffee and staring out at the fog over the river. Over a third cup, it suddenly struck me: you are not the virus; the virus is not you. I had been looking at you through an AIDS scrim, my vision baffled by the virus. Suddenly you stood before me for the first time, just you, no longer shadowed by your viral load, and I so liked who I saw. The virus had already claimed far too many, far too much. How much a victory was I to allow it? Together, if it worked out, we could snatch something out of its fanged trap. A couple of affectionate fucks, at the least. Maybe some companionship for a time?

I called you up. "Join me for dinner Tuesday night at the house of two friends of mine. They want to meet you."

"Tuesday night. . . Tuesday night. . ."

"Cancel it," I said. "They have a hot tub. I'll pick you up at 6:00."

This would be your final exam, your last audition.

You were charming at dinner. My friends were dazzled, the old queens. They were wicked enough to set out escargot picks with nothing to use them on, just to see what you would do with yours.

"Where are the snails?" you asked. You brought the right wine.

After dinner we all got into the hot tub naked, clunking our wine glasses down on the redwood decking. The air was arctic, wisps of gauze wreathing up from the dark water and whipping away in the wind. They went to bed, enjoining us to turn off the jets when we left.

I slipped through the water to sit beside you, my hand on your thigh. No more tests. You had passed them all, even the physical I gave you as you undressed. You were not perfect. You had no butt to speak of. Alas. Your legs were lean and roped with standout veins. So much else was splendid: your small nipples in aureolae large as bronze coins, for instance. Your penis was luscious.

We sat together in this warm inland sea, Aphrodite rising. The winter-chapped hands of a palm tree creaked arthritically above us in the wind. The powdered face of the moon faded and formed, an old coquette among clouds.

The bedroom light went off in a distant corner of the house behind you. I whispered in the whorl of your ear. You darted your tongue lightly over your lower lip, closed your eyes. Your kisses were always as ardent as this first one.

We left, damp and shivering, by the garden gate at the side of the house. The fog had lowered. We would light a fire in the black granite hearth of your living room, your arms and chest golden in the glow as we lay together in that warmth. I would spend the night, first of so many.

MARKS

"Are you coming?" you called from the bedroom.

I stood in the doorway. You were in bed, your face turned towards me.

"What takes you so long in the bathroom?" you asked.

"One must labor to be beautiful," I replied.

You swept the sheet aside. I slid in next to you, sidled up to your naked warmth.

"Sleepy?"

"Read me a poem."

Your breathing grew regular and heavy. I finished the poem, laid the book aside, watched you doze. You opened your eyes, the blue of snow in moonlight.

"Mmmm," you murmured.

I brushed your hair back.

You turned and looked up at my bedroom ceiling.

"What's that?" you asked, pointing at a scratched mark about the diameter of a quarter where the paint had been pulled away.

"A previous boyfriend did that."

"He should have trimmed his toenails," you said.

"Perhaps," I laughed, "but the explanation's more lame. One evening Mark stuck up adhesive glow-in-the-dark stars on this ceiling while I was fixing dinner. When we went to bed later and I turned out the light, the ceiling spangled like the night sky. 'It's just like we're boy scouts camping out in the backyard and buggering in our tent,' Mark said. 'And that's where you'll be sleeping if you do any more decorating around here,' I told him."

"What happened to Mark?"

"Oh, he went the way of all my old boyfriends—fuck and be gone, out the door, fast and without fuss.

"I'd fuss," you said.

AIDS had as yet left no marks on your body. I wondered what I would do on detecting a purple blotch on your chest or a white bloom of thrush at the corner of your mouth.

In the morning, after the sex, its slick wetness and raw, earthy odors, after you had showered, shaved, dressed, gone to work, I went back into the bedroom from the breakfast table littered with your scanned morning paper and the chipped blue bowl with your half-eaten oatmeal. I started to make the bed. "Such a good fuck," I mused. I started to plump the pillows. But I hesitated on seeing, in the divot where your head had lain, one golden hair coiled like a question mark.

OUT OF THE BLUE

I

"Mendocino Inn. This is Kirk. How may I assist you?"

I knew he was gay.

"I'm calling about the weekend special advertised in my local paper: two nights at the Inn, a complementary dinner for two, two tickets to a play. . . ."

"Good deal, isn't it? Off season. So what paper did you catch our ad in? *Bay Area Reporter*?"

"*Mom Guess What!*"

"Excremento! Used to live there till the nasty pneumie got me. . . the bad kind. Flat on my back for weeks I was with no one on top! Couldn't draw in enough breath to talk … or even to suck, if you can believe it! Yes, we can accommodate you, but I need to ask you a few questions."

"Shoot."

"Oh <u>baby</u>! Let's not be premature. Okay, are you both over twenty-one, have a major credit card—other than your gay card, of course?"

"What?! Yes."

"Good. And the nature of your relationship?"

"I beg your pardon?"

Sigh. "Husband? Partner? Lover? Boyfriend? Date? Trick? . . . Trade?"

I was silent.

"Hustler?   Boy-toy?   Man-of-your-dreams-for-this-weekend-only?   Hamburger-while-you're-waiting-for-steak?"

"Now wait a minute."

"Look, Mary, I'm just trying to put you in the best accommodations for your situation. Now work with me."

"Date," I blurted.

"Then the garden suite, of course. Just leave it all to Kirk—that's K-I-R-Q-U-E."

"Really?"

Pause. Imagined eye roll.

"Oh, it'll be the most romantic weekend ever! Trust me! Flowers, food. . . .By the way, skip the play. Downer! How long have you and . . .er. . . ."

"Dore."

"Like 'revolving door'?"

"Now look . . . ."

"How long have you guys been 'dating'?"

"So what time is check-in?"

"Not long, then. We'll see you Friday evening any time after 3:00. You're booked. Drive safely."

Click.

That evening: "Dore, I made the reservations for this weekend in Mendocino with some caricature called Kirk. All he did was camp."

"Confirm. Definitely."

The next morning I called again.

"Mendocino Inn. This is Kirk."

"Kirk, this is Lu from Sacramento. I'm calling to confirm our reservation for this weekend."

"Lu: you do not have to ring me up every five minutes. I am a professional. I am anal about details. You're anal too, I'll bet. Hostelry is my calling. The three of us have a hot little date this weekend in the garden suite."

Click.

II

"About time you boys got here," said the young man behind the reception desk. The clock above him read 7:22. "You've kept us in suspense for hours. We didn't know when to expect your arrival." He glanced sternly from wristwatch to us to wristwatch.

"You must be Kirk," I said.

"And you must be Dore!" he said, not glancing in my direction, appraising you, face to feet, feet to face.

Scarcely twenty-five, Kirk looked as if he had just fought off the AIDS pneumocystis he had earlier alluded to. His coral shirt, buttoned at the throat with a ruby starburst pin and falling in loose folds down to his thighs, was an apparent attempt to disguise the body gauntness one could read in his face. He wore tight black jeans ending in pointy black come-fuck-me boots. He was in the last stages of cute: his spiked hair flared copper at the tips; his eyes were large and green and moist; wispy patches of whiskers over and under his lips testified to hopeless attempts to coax out a goatee at the borders of hollow cheeks.

"Here, fill this in," he said, pushing a registration card vaguely in my direction, still smiling fetchingly at you.

While I wrote my driver's license and address, a chinless, fleshy projection of Kirk in thirty more years (if he was very lucky) opened a door from a back office and came behind the desk. "Wally," he said, "when these guests have registered, let's close out the cash drawer. I'll drop the bag off at night deposit on my way home."

"It's <u>Kirk</u>," Kirk insisted in a level, dangerous voice.

"This month," the older man said.

Our suite was the upper floor of a new extension built at the back of the gardens. We lit a fire in the sitting area and flipped the lights off. The firelight glowed through the curtains enclosing the bed alcove, veining the folds of the blue counterpane in gold like a sheet of lapis lazuli.

The phone rang.

"Is everything to your satisfaction?" Kirk asked. "Do you require anything? Pillows plumped? Bed turned down? Additional towels? Champagne? Chocolates? More firewood? Coffee? Tea? Us three?"

"Thank you for everything, Kirk," I said. "It's a beautiful room. We're very happy."

"Lucky little you."

Click.

III

We woke to sunlight and bird trill and the spiced odor of the wood fire, embers now, and the distant respirations of the ocean. I took photographs of you tangled in white sheets, laughing, protesting. We filled the Jacuzzi, lay entwined in water energized, white foam over blue sea salts. I loved the tautness of you, your sharp planes, angularities. Our movements sloshed water onto the floor.

At breakfast you scanned the menu, then tossed it down and glanced out the window. Sunlight splashed into the dining room. I looked up at the pressed-tin ceiling, painted so often that its pattern had lost its crispness. "I am happy alone," I reflected, "a lean, wiry contentment." I glanced at you appraising. The light shifted: I saw only you, your outline crisp as paper. In this sudden concentration, I glimpsed your merit, from which all your acts and thoughts branched: a distilled grace, a sweetness boned in strength. Through this rift, you shone essential. Your HIV evanesced for me as a defining trait. Once and for all.

IV

On Mendocino's main street, we entered a second-story shop up an interior stairway. The left wall of the stairwell offered a levitation of planets and stars against a saturated blue. In the same blue on the right side, a gray whale breached. Fish swam. In the shop, you pushed a jade planchette over a Ouija board. I plucked the strings of several Aeolian harps of varying sizes until told not to by the shop owner, an ancient lady wavering in aquamarine, her white hair stapled with shell barrettes: "Human fingers untune them. Here!" She put several harps in open windows: "Let the breath of the Spirit play over them without the discord we make. Listen! This one sings in the voice of the sea!"

The shop door whooshed open to a shiver of silver bells.

"Waaaa-lllleeee!" lilted the old woman.

"It's Kirrr-irrrk!" lilted Kirk. He plopped a blue mailbag on the counter and turned and beamed at you, head raked at a coy angle.

You were idly flipping through a deck of Tarot cards.

"Do you see a young man with green eyes and fabulous hair flaming into your future?" Kirk asked in a stage-whisper, sidling up to you.

"No he does not," I called from across the shop.

"Wasn't talking to you, Mary," said Kirk without turning to me.

"And stop calling me Mary, Wally," I said.

Kirk scanned the cards you were laying out. "Here's the King of Wands. That's you, of course: fair hair, blue eyes, successful in business, a professional man. Sensible. Stubborn at times. You know your mind."

You laughed and laid out several more cards. I joined you.

"Just look at all those cups tumbling out! Here's the six: marriage of mind and body and spirit. Next is the Ace of Cups: the beginning of love and happiness."

You laid out more cards.

"More cups! Cupids and doves and hearts and gooey desserts shared with the same fork, blah, blah, blah. Okay, here's the Knight of Cups reversed: perhaps transition. Struggle? Conflict? The two of wands follows, though: partnership, cooperation, someone willing to give assistance. Very lucky sequence!"

You flipped out three more cards.

"Umhmm, here he is at last, late on the scene," Kirk said, glancing at me. He picked up the Page of Pentacles, fanned himself with it, tossed it down. "Fits, mostly. Dark hair, near-sighted, contrary." He appraised me grudgingly, looked away. "Definitely not young and pretty."

You began to gather up the strewn cards.

"Deal a few of the Majors," Kirk suggested, pointing to a deck beside the one you squared on the red silk scarf they rested on.

The old lady tottered up. "Wally here thinks he's the High Priestess," she whispered to me. "She does seem to surface somewhere whenever he reads. But actually he's the Knight of Swords: he has good intentions, but he can be fractious. He's good at the Tarot, though," she added proudly. "Taught him everything he knows."

"No, thank you," you said, seeing me eye my watch.

"Oh, really you should," said the old lady. "How about he read you?" she added, turning to me.

"Well, ta-ta!" said Kirk immediately. "Enough of this bliss! Duty calls."

"No rest for the wicked," I added.

V

You needed food to take with your medications—a bright pink, green, blue mosaic of hope. "You are what you eat," you said, downing a handful of pills. "So I've become a Walgreens."

After lunch, we ambled out through salt meadows, grasshoppers ticking in the tall grasses, until we came up to the high rocks of the Mendocino Headlands. I scrambled after you up a tumble, scanning for sandy footholds, scraped fingers fumbling in the boulder flanks. It was a slippery, arduous climb. It was dangerous to have tried it in sandals.

Topping the rocks, out of breath, I was dissolved in a blue rush! Before me was an infinite azure plane: No motion. No moorings. No horizons, either of sea or sky. In that dizzy instant, I tottered. I feared I would fall from the uneven boulder I teetered on into that blue void. And then you were beside me, your arm around my waist, drawing me back. You were looking, not at the sea, but at me, your blue eyes anchoring me again. You leaned into me.

I knew then, on those rocks over that blue abstraction, that I would never be the same again, that I had never felt this grounding in another human being before, this radical life-shift.

Now here I stood before heaven, an apostate. I had always believed love to be a necessary fiction evolved in heterosexuals to bond a man and a woman for the rearing of children. When gay men "fell in love," they fell victim to a heterosexual infection. Their minds, fevered from some straight contagion, failed to realize their gay gift, its promiscuous freedoms. But this counterproof had come suddenly upon me out of the blue. What had I fallen into here?

My affection for men in the past had always been tentative, a withholding. I had kept my running shoes by the door. Now this! I could not yet apply the word, though it hovered in the blue air.

VI

Soon the sun began to brood. It was time for you to have your nap, to take your meds. Reluctantly, we walked back through the meadows to the village. The grasshoppers had hushed, as if in a waiting rapture. The hotel gardens had grown sage in the waning light.

Inside, the room was dark and too warm. I opened the window. I spied Kirk across the garden sitting on the steps at the back entrance to the hotel kitchens, spindly arms extended behind to brace him, his head cocked at a fetching angle, shadows deepening the collapse of his cheeks. He was staring at a young kitchen worker, dark, tattooed, taut as a knife blade, who had come out into the dusk to smoke a cigarette. He held it between thumb and forefinger, ignoring Kirk.

I drew the gauze sheers against this vision of fruitless desiring. A listless breeze shifted them, mingling rose and geranium with the faint scent of wood smoke lingering in the room.

"The French call this time of day 'l'heure bleu,'" I said.

"I can see why," you said.

"Are you blue in mood?"

"I'm happy," you said.

We lay down in the bed with our clothes on. I dozed but woke soon, listening in the neutral light to the blended murmurs of the sea, your sleeping, a few birds chirping in garden trees. I woke again in the dark and went to sit in a chair facing the bed. I watched you sleeping. It came to me then that you were the only person I had ever imagined spending the rest of my life with. For the first time ever, the word "love" clicked into my consciousness as if it fitted there.

You opened your eyes. You tried to focus, looking at me with a frown. You arched your long back, your arms up over your head. You stared at me for a moment. Then, as you reached to click the light on, you smiled, and the light flooded the blue bed alcove.

"Come here," you said—but I was already on my way.

VII

The dining room of the Mendocino Inn was nearly empty, the hour being early. We sat at a table for two against an old-brick wall, candlelight warm on white linens.

"Smart little cocktails, gentlemen?"

"You!" I said.

"Just who did you expect? Judy Garland's dead. In case you hadn't noticed, I'm a working girl. You don't think I'm able to afford my glamorous life from the pittance I earn standing at the reception desk, now do you?" Kirk fanned his free hand before us. A diamond and emerald dinner ring gleamed on his middle finger. "This little bijou did not arrive in a Cracker Jack box." He winked at me: "Want to be my sugar daddy?"

You rested your forehead in your hand and laughed.

"Don't encourage him," I snapped.

"I'll give you gentlemen a little longer with the menu. Meanwhile, why doesn't Kirk bring you two extra-dry martinis and an iddy snacky, okee-dokee?"

"How did you know we drink martinis?" I demanded.

"I'm also the maid. You should see me in my little black shift and lace apron. Very A-line Dior. It hitches up over my backside when I have to scour the tub—because certain people just have to use the bath salts."

Kirk frowned at me.

"Extra-dry martinis because Kirk couldn't find any vermouth in your room," he continued. "And you drink Bombay Sapphire—unless you've funneled the cheap stuff into that enchanting blue bottle?"

"It's the real thing, Kirk," you said.

"I know that, gorgeous," Kirk winked. "I took a nip."

When he had left, I whispered to you, "I am tired of playing straight man to Kirk."

Over my shoulder I heard a snort: "<u>You</u>?" A straight man? Puh-leeese, Mary."

We studied the menu. The martinis were perfect. I forgave Kirk everything.

"How's the salmon, Kirk?" I asked when he returned to take our order.

He shrugged. "It's fresh."

"The pork chops?" you asked.

"Oh, _my_!" Kirk trilled, stepping back from the table, his jeweled hand flat against his chest. "Excellent choice, sir!"

Kirk clearly enjoyed flourishing the silver warming dome away, for the pork chops were actually a small pork roast glazed in a fruit and root-vegetable corona, the whole a Dutch still life. My Spartan salmon in caper sauce turned appetizer, we shared your dish.

At times fortune conspires to prove the possibility of perfection in this fallen world. Other than Kirk and his baroque approval of you, I do not recall one flat moment during this weekend. Would I have fallen in love with you then had we had a broken water hose in the car on the way up, the two of us standing at the border of the dripping woods, the car hood raised, the motor hissing an angry spume into the miles of darkness? Or if the inn had lost our reservation, was booked, had checked us into a damp little room in a dilapidated old motel in Fort Bragg plunked down next to a trailer park, no ocean in sight? If I had fallen at the rocks of the Mendocino Headlands, as almost happened, had broken a wrist, say, the two of us deliberating what to do, stranded together in a strange, uncertain place?

Instead of disaster that day, we were favored, proof against distress. Never has the world been for me so receptive, so happy-tripping over itself to please.

VIII

After dinner and against Kirk's repeated advice, we went to the play on our complimentary tickets, the Goetz dramatization of Gide's *The Immoralists*, directed by a former colleague of mine from Cal State who, having just retired from the drama department, somehow got the fantastic notion to stage an early homosexual play for the edification of a yuppie Republican village. As I watched the scantly attended play, I got to thinking of all the human ruin resulting from being gay among cultures which condemned it. What a weary struggle for us throughout post-Hellenic history—the hangings and burnings and stonings, all the shrouded secrets and shame and exile and changed pronouns, the agonized self-crucifixions, the destruction of others unfortunate in their attachments to us, lost as we were in our own fearful hiding from ourselves and from those we were supposed to hold dear. Where is our rage, our gay fury at this? The unraveled lives flickering on that shabby stage compressed our sad history before us in the darkness. And now, with gay liberation a real possibility for us, along comes AIDS. Were we ever meant to win? Maybe Kirk was right in advising us not to attend this play.

It was good to come out of that cramp at the end of the play to walk into a night glazed with stars. We approached the edge of town, behind us a few dim streetlights. We could hear the booming of the sea beyond. The wind sang through the sea grasses; it whirled the myriads of hard, bright stars.

There at the confluence of land and sea and luminous night sky, we stood just through the doorway of our time together. Stars and grasses, the ocean deep breathing, the glancing winds were all of a piece. We were entering a glimmering darkness together, lost heirs come home at last.

We cut through the midnight lobby on the way back to our suite off the gardens. There, behind the desk, stood Kirk. He gazed at us without speaking. His hair bristled in points of coppery flame.

In the room, the fire had been kindled. On a low side table a silver ice bucket braced a bottle of champagne. Two crystal flutes gleamed in the firelight. A note on blue paper lay propped against a plate of chocolates:

Love is everything!

Derek
(formerly Kirk, nee Wally)

BRACKETS

Oddly, in spite of having been a love-atheist, I was always a romantic, all gush and coo. I used to fuss over the few tricks that I allowed to return, after heroic sex-a-thons. I did everything but fall in love with them. I played music I thought they would like, offered them food and good wine. Set out flowers and used fresh linens in anticipation of bedding them again. You get the picture. . . .

You, on the other hand, were not romantic. An anecdote will illustrate: We visited a few times with my friends George and Neil (drag name: "Iona Doublewide") at their trailer home in the Nevada desert just outside of Reno. You liked staying there enough that you put up with their three big dogs, dissuading their drooling overtures by guiding them away with your foot.

George and Neil preferred to visit us in Sacramento but were for a time housebound: George had contracted cryptosporidiosis, apparently during a business trip to Milwaukee, and had to have a shunt implanted to infuse himself with a potent new drug to combat the bloody diarrhea, severe and chronic, that had earlier killed so many immune-compromised gay men with crypto, a severe bacterial bowel infection, his type originally found only in the guts of sheep. George had lost 63 pounds, his skin draping over the bones of his arms. We could visit them only because George's doctor had determined that he could no longer pass on this vicious gut parasite. Things looked promising: George had re-gained 28 of the lost pounds since beginning the infusions.

So far, Neil was holding his own after a bout with PCP the year before. But it was Neil who would die first, a year later, demented from a sudden savage onslaught of toxoplasmosis.

George snapped the photograph of you and me toasting each other with martinis at sunset on their deck overlooking miles of empty sagebrush. The hills backing us in the photo are mottled in mauve and cream.

The night we took that photo, George and I were preparing supper in the kitchen just after the last light had leached from the hills. You and Neil were discussing the stock market in the living room. I was busy at the sink getting up a salad. A brilliance flared into the window, as if a lighthouse had sent its sudden beam through it. Startled, I glanced up to see, over the crest of a brown hill, a full moon bobbing up, enormous in a violet sky. George and I watched it untether itself from the hill and float free, its craters tarnished silver.

I rushed into the living room, dogs jumping up at my hurry, and insisted that you come with me to see something breathtaking. The dogs were game—frisking, tails wagging. You followed me, demurring. "What?" you said. When I gestured to the moon, you batted me on the upper arm. "That old thing?" you said. "I've seen it a hundred times before."

You turned to go back into the living room. I grabbed you around the waist. "Oh no you don't," I protested. "You do not turn your back on this. You are going to look at that moon with me." You groused about venturing out in the cold. I flicked the kitchen light off and led you to the back deck.

"It's cold," you said. "Have you looked enough?"

"This must be my magic," I sighed. "I'm a moonchild. The sun is your star."

Back in the house, I listened to you conversing with Neil about the NASDAQ. When I looked out again, the moon had dimmed a murky yellow and slipped off out of range of the window.

"George," I said, "this with Dore has gotten serious."

"Serious! Is this really you talking? You're having a stroke, right?"

"We're so different, but it feels right."

"Look," said George, "no one was more surprised than me when I fell for Neil. I would never have thought he was my type. Here's how I read the attraction between you and Dore, other than the sex, which you attest is consummate: You complement. Dore's fire and earth. You're air and water."

"Earth I can see, but Dore as fire? He's not at all combustible. Well, he does fire up into a perfect conflagration while I'm licking his . . . ."

"Whoa! Keep something back, will you? But to the point: Look at your separate houses. Yours is all air and water with its high ceilings, its play of light from the river. Every time I come to your house I throw myself on your window seat to look at the clouds pushing through the windows in your living room. You like mirrors and glass and silver. Now take Dore's house. . . ."

"I get it now," I interrupted. "It's horizontal, ranch style, with cherry wood in the kitchen and brown paisley chairs grouped before a black-granite hearth. His house looks out on a closed garden walled by redwoods."

"Like I said, all fire and earth."

"Our personalities tend that way too," I added. "I tend to storm; he calms and settles."

We peered into the living room. "Look at those two," George laughed. "Anyone would think they belong together."

"Like you and me?" I asked.

"That'd be a BEYOND no," George grimaced.

In looking back, I cannot explain how I could fall in love with you after so many years of denial that love could be real for gay men. And to love you so quickly after meeting you. George thought I allowed myself to let you in because at some level I suspected that our time together was to be condensed. He may be right, though I think my opening to you had a more indirect, more convoluted impetus: Shortly before meeting you, I was introduced by the AIDS Foundation to Gordon, a violinist who had given up his apartment, car, and symphony chair to move back home with his parents. He no longer left his bedroom: Kaposi sarcoma lesions, some raised and textured, others smooth as leather, covered his face, skeletal now and fringed with limp, colorless wisps of hair where he was not able to shave. Internal K S lesions had invaded his lungs and spleen. Herpes blisters, some in colonies seven inches across, covered his forearms and legs. When I met him, he looked like a Giacometti standing figure.

Gordon was a movie fanatic: He wanted to watch his favorite films a final time with someone to talk with about them. I was there for that, having put on my AIDS Foundation application my own love for film.

One afternoon he called and asked me to come over. When I entered his room, he hoisted himself up painfully from his chair. His pajama bottoms fell to the floor, pooling at his feet. He weighed 106 pounds. I helped him right them over his diaper.

"I wanted to say goodbye," he said. "My doctor says I'll go sometime next week. I'm ready. I can't eat. I can't drink anymore. Even water goes right through me or comes back up and I choke on it. I now have lesions in my stomach and adrenal glands."

"I'll miss you," I said.

"I caught AIDS from my lover who left me as soon as I got sick. I was poisonously bitter about that for a long time, living alone, not wanting to see anyone, gorging on anger and hurt. Closed way down in a dark place. Then one day my parents barged into my apartment without warning or even knocking and pleaded with me to move back home, to be, as they put it, where I was loved. Pretty moving of them when some parents are afraid even to go near their AIDS-infected sons. So I opened up enough to let them in again. They'll be there at the end with me here in my old bedroom, rounding the circle. I'll be buried out of the church I went to as a boy. They'll play a recording of me bowing my violin to conclude the service—one time more before I have to trade my violin in for a harp. All I've ever done with my life is make music. Pretty harmless, right?"

Perhaps it was Gordon who provided the roundabout connection with my opening to you when I did. He showed me how bracketed and locked a life can be. Mine especially: my brackets have always been closed tight. Gordon's at the end opened. I felt the rightness in that. Your brackets opened out for me in a similar way toward the end. You knew you were dying long before I realized it. I somehow had the grace to enter that opening you made for me, thereby releasing my own life constraints. I remember Gordon with gratitude.

Later that night, as you slept beside me in the Nevada desert, wind whirring over the corrugated metal siding of the trailer, I counted our bracket expansions: I took you to opera at San Francisco's War Memorial; you took me to Broadway musicals. I read the articles you clipped for me from the Wall Street Journal; you listened to me read poetry and joined me in watching foreign films on PBS, after, that is, we watched the Nightly Business Report. I learned from you that love places one in those regions of the world previously closed to him. It wedges open brackets, widening spaces in life a person might never have entered by himself. Love alleges that living is more wondrous and inexhaustible for both partners than either had previously suspected on his own. The test of love is not infatuated exhilaration, though it is nice when that accompanies love. The test of love is growth: does love make both partners better, wider, more open, more alive?

You were not romantic. Perhaps that was for the best. You spared me the hollow and self-conscious romantic gestures that would have spooked me, especially in our early days together. We were to make life larger for each other, especially when so many lives all around us were contracting, bracketing, flickering out in a Losing Time.

PARLEYING

By rights we should not have been able to sit outside, but it had been an unusually warm day in early March, enticing robins to bob and race along the trails by the river. Pink blurs of wild plum glimmered through the bare willow thickets fringing the river. We were drinking martinis, triangular glasses glinting in the darkening light.

On an impulse, I reached over and took your hand: "I'm in love with you."

You left your hand in mine.

"I could never have said this before. I can't believe I'm saying it now."

Several moments passed.

"I just wish I had met you twenty years earlier," you said quietly.

"But twenty years ago neither of us would have been ready."

Again a long silence.

"I'm thinking about my health."

When we first sat in the frail evening sunlight, you glowed in well-being: your eyes a clear azure; your lower lip full and bronzy pink.

"You're on Invirase and other new drugs. People are living longer now. Even those who have picked out their caskets are returning to life, like Lazarus called back. The last memorial service I went to was almost two weeks ago."

"The doctor told me today that my few remaining T-cells can't stand up against the highest viral load ever recorded in his office. How we all eye each other in that waiting room, sizing up what the virus is doing to us. . . ."

"But they'll get it right, the drug cocktail. They just need to figure out the right combinations." You were on your second re-configured pill regimen. You carried an ice pack to keep your meds chilled. A pill case with a beeper rang the times you were to take them.

How singular it must have been for you to hear of the virus's rampage on the very day I would first declare my love for you. I did not then join the two messages in my own mind as you must have: the new lover is always an arrant egoist, centered in his own wonder. This early March day marked for us an odd merger: my moment of heightened feeling with your grim new awareness of the relentless viral onslaught. You showed me a dim swirling in the distance. But I saw detours before we reached that roadblock. I could not share your urgency then.

I do not know how to write about beginning to love. Most people learned about loving long before I did. This I think I know: love is at first more about the self than about the other. The lover is in renewal. At least I was. New love impels one to throw out and discard, to make donations to good will. So inward a renewal for me was loving that you did not even have to know you were loved. The lover makes himself new, his world novel.

As a new lover, I was forever monitoring feelings and perceptions. I inventoried emotions, fascinated by the shifting hues and shadows. That is the reason sex between us in those early days was so insistent, never frequent enough. In lovemaking, I could for a time step into the sway of your stride. I could know you then when you were most open to me.

"I want us to be monogamous," you said out of the darkness.

"Monogamy is for breeders," I said disdainfully. "Gay men were not made to promise never to touch another man. A quick blow job at the Steamworks in Berkeley on a solo Friday night? So what? Emotional monogamy, definitely. But sexual monogamy evolved to protect straight child-bearers against outside disruptions in family life. What has that to do with us?"

"Stop talking," you said. "I don't need a lecture on gay sexual politics, especially not right now."

I waited out the silence.

You sighed. "Just don't let me ever hear of anything."

I know now, I thought, that love exists. And I was happy. We were bold lovers that night.

What can I not know? Much: Why did love come to me during the plague and with you, already stricken? Why was our love plighted in impermanence? Was George right? Did I allow myself to love at last because at some level I knew that AIDS would lift from me the burden of love grown bald and corpulent and querulous? Because I surmised we could thus avoid the love-crippling compromises most lovers eventually come to make over time?

Did you love me? One can never really know if one is loved. This uncertainty joins the clutter of unknowable things jumbled together in the black-lacquered drawers of the unconscious, useless and vital things all tangled up together. You told me you had never been in love before. You had dated someone once, for about six months, but you had soon found him bland.

Did you love me? For the first months of our time together, you insisted regularly that you could not find anything wrong with me. I lost patience at last: "I'm tired of interviewing for this lover position," I finally said. "Do I have it or not? And can I earn tenure?"

Whenever I told you I loved you—infrequently, even after that first twilit time—you responded, automatically, "Love you <u>too</u>!" with a lilt on the adverb, sounding like some teenager in a mini-skirt saying goodbye to her girlfriends after a day shopping together at the mall. But one day, months later, I called to check in with you from a lonely hotel room in a suburb of San Francisco, oppressed by its fake Biedermeier furniture, its tired mauve bedspread. For some reason I paused. A beat or two passed. You filled the small stillness: "I love you."

There it was—you first, no lilt.

"Surprised you?"

"Thrilled me."

DEATH VALLEY

I

A green morning in April: the world is wet from an early shower, but a pert young sun is winning out, pinching the puckered butts of weighty clouds slipping past in offended dignity. A scrub jay screeches at a mockingbird, a doughty warrior who gives as good as it gets. A ginger cat watches for casualties, hunched under a purple azalea.

I am waiting for you and your sister Bonnie to arrive. The RV pulls up, portly as a church lady in sensible shoes. Bonnie is proud of her rig: a 27-foot Class A Winnebago, the fully loaded 1992 deluxe model with the big motor option and customized air ride—in short, a lesbian dream-mobile.

The three of us are setting out on a Spring Break road trip I suggested—over the Sierra at Tahoe and down Highway 395 to Death Valley, then on to Las Vegas. You and I will fly back to Sacramento on Easter Sunday, and Bonnie will continue on to Palm Springs for the Dinah Shore golf classic and attendant lesbian frolics.

I grab my bag and walk out through the courtyard to the street. You are standing outside of the RV watching me approach. Whenever I see you, I have a feeling equivalent to walking home after the last day of spring term, my grades all turned in, September way off down a corridor of blue summer air.

Bonnie emerges from the back of the rig. She is stout and short, chesty from years of heavy smoking. Her gray, wavy hair is cropped close. She has fine gray eyes, the bright color of winter fog thinning before a sun gaining in confidence. She describes herself as a "soft butch." She gives me a glance, up and down, unaccustomed as she is to your having boyfriends.

"So you're the man my brother has been talking so much about." I do not know how to answer this.

We climb aboard. You staked a claim to the couch and insisted that I take one of the swivel chairs that served as front seats. We swayed in a ponderous lope up Highway 50 towards Tahoe, semis whizzing past us to the left and right. The RV dipped and jived up and down hills like a genial but not overly bright mare, eager to please but too old and clumsy to gallop.

Bonnie and I peered at each other out of the corners of our eyes. I looked back at you. You looked up, abstracted, from the map, which I also needed now to find my way in a world you had reconfigured.

"Take the Camino exit, Bon," you said. "Lunch time. I have to take my pills."

I had heard about Ruby's. You and your friends from work occasionally drove out there for drinks and dinner on the weekends when they had a band and redneck dancing. Ruby's reminded me of barbecue dives in the dusty, ramshackle hill towns outside of Austin, Texas. We graduate students used to drive out in our dented Pintos and Valiants and Falcons to watch the locals two-step on Saturday evenings. We would suck down greasy barbecued ribs and stagecoach beans and get shit-faced on longneck Lone Stars and later have to pull off the highway onto gravel side roads to sleep it off when our weaving threatened to end us up in the headlight glare of a cattle truck barreling down on us in a spume of gravel and dust.

Bonnie pulled the rig onto Ruby's unpaved parking lot. Most of the vehicles there were pickups with gun racks spanning their back windows. The far corner of the lot was reserved for fifth-wheels and RVs. We jostled over ruts to that corner. Bonnie suddenly braked her RV and stared hard. A duplicate of her rig materialized before us: the exact same make, the same model and upgrades. But this rig was a reflection in a twisted mirror. It was like a chance meeting of identical twins long separated, one flush with success, the other one beaten down by lousy luck and bad choices. Rust pocked its side panels. Its windshield was a scatter of glass spider webs. Its bent engine grille framed a bug-spattered placard indicating the rig belonged to "The Dwindle's."

Bonnie parked her rig reluctantly next to its dilapidated duplicate in the only spot left on the lot. When we got out, we peered cautiously through the bent blind slats of the side window. Grease splotches blossomed over the lavender florals of the wallpaper. The sprung oven door was tied shut to the microwave handle by a piece of frayed rope.

Suddenly a gray Chihuahua leapt up into the window space, teeth bared, the fur around its snout pure white. It more coughed than barked, but still it startled us. That did it for Bonnie. She plodded grimly towards Ruby's and twanged open the screen door.

Ruby's was aptly named: the walls of the bar and dining rooms were clad in rough-planed redwood boards. Pale sunlight struggled through windows curtained in stained red gingham, and the bluish air inside was rich with the smells of roasting and frying and smoking and barbecuing meat. Carnivore heaven. Heads of all creatures horned and hoofed were mounted on red plywood shields. This snug lair in the hills offered a grotesque inversion of the Ark. A dusty fox, forefoot lifted warily, stared at us with glass eyes from a ledge above our table.

You had pre-sorted your pills into daily portions. No escape: AIDS followed us, like an unpleasant odor. You opened a packet filled with the rainbow reminders of the battle being waged. "Better living through chemicals," you cracked, and downed a handful in two gulps, the lexicon of desperate hope: at various times interleukin 2, AL721, AZT, ddI, ddC, d4T, 3TC, Septra, Bactrim, pentamidine, foscarnet, acyclovir, invirase, eventually norvir, crixivan, other drugs. This chemical cocktail constantly shifted. You and others were essentially lab rats for desperate scientists looking for some way to stop the virus. You had begun to take the protease inhibitor Invirase, then new on the scene and, according to your doctor, the most promising med yet. Your breath always smelled of the pharmaceuticals that suffused your system. You had been taking many of these drugs serially for so long that the virus was now in near-continuous mutation.

Lunch over, we skirted puddles in the parking lot and approached the rig. "Hey!" yelled Bonnie at the couple cupping their hands over her side window and scoping out our rig through the open blind slats. "Can I help you?"

"Your rigged? Know you're happy with it!" said a frail, elderly man turning to face us. "I'm Hap. Hap Dwindle. And this here's my greater half." He gestured to the hefty woman hulking by his side. "Her name's Peaches. Peaches Dwindle. Sweet and juicy like a peach." Peaches cuffed him on the upper arm, sending him staggering.

Hap flattened his nose against the window and peered into the rig again. "Just like us's," he said rheumily, turning to face us again. Bonnie glared at the smeared window.

Hap had eyes the color of wet newspaper and a bald pate spattered with age spots. Peaches stood stolid beside him, smiling, her teeth butter yellow.

"Where ya'll headed?" asked Hap.

"Through Tahoe to 395," I said. "On to Vegas."

Bonnie turned and frowned at me, her lips tight.

Meanwhile, Peaches was walking to her rig, her buttocks tussling together like two pigs struggling in a gunny sack. She cracked open her rig door and the Chihuahua jumped through the frame where the screen should have been. He lifted an arthritic hind leg against the front tire of Bonnie's rig.

"Git!" Bonnie said.

"Come on over here, li'l Dopey," Peaches said. "This is Dopey Dwindle. He come by his name in Disneyland."

"Like a speck of coffee? Got some heating from last night," added Hap.

"We're behind schedule," snapped Bonnie, unlocking the RV. As we jounced out of the parking lot, we passed the Dwindles, grinning and waving at us.

The several pints of India Pale Ale I had had with lunch soon kicked in, so you sat up front with Bonnie and navigated. I dozed, listening to you and Bonnie. The conversations of those who are intimate go low, nearly inflectionless. In the last months of your life, I heard us talk this way while sitting together in your doctor's waiting room.

The RV labored up a steep incline, its thermometer needle inching toward the red zone. Bonnie pulled off at a turnout. We huddled by the side of the road, kicking with our sneakers at snow crusts lapping over thin rivulets of melt.

We heard a dull clanking noise and turned just in time to see the Dwindles speed by in a whir of blue exhaust, a lawn chair too loosely tied to the back banging against a bumper. Their horn blatted the first bars of "The Eyes of Texas Are upon You." Dopey rested two paws against the rear window, his head wobbling like a bobble-doll.

II

Towards evening we lumbered downhill into Bridgeport with its lake elongating northeastward. Bonnie parked the rig at a hook-up in an RV park. A wiry little man with eyes set close to his nose directed us through arm movements and a flashlight into our crumbled asphalt pad with the elaborate precision of a runway jockey guiding a jetliner into its bay.

After dinner, Bonnie went into the back bedroom. A light came on, rosy through the acetate curtain. I heard her turn pages in her western and grind a cigarette out in an ashtray.

I took you by the hand and led you outside. The night sky flared with stars. And then there it was, what I had led you out to see: a blotch of drifting greenish light, an unraveled glow—the comet Hale-Bopp suspended above black ridges. It had taken 2500 years to get here; no one would see it again for another 2500 years. We stood for a moment, side by side, in wonder. Then you shifted behind me, wrapped your arms around me, your cheek coming to rest against the side of my head.

As I gazed on that comet, it came to me that love was gravity, that I was grounded at last among these stars, these interruptions in all this emptiness. I looked at Hale-Bopp and the star fields it floated through. You filled the loneliness I had not realized was there before you.

"That there's a clear sign in heaven of the end times," croaked Hap, materializing out of the darkness. He cleared his throat.

You jumped away from me.

"I know the Rapture's soon upon us 'cause most mornings I feel giddy in my bones. Are you saved in the blood of the blessed assurance? Don't much look like it to me. There's yet time," he added, peering from me to you, one eye wide open, the other nearly closed.

"You leave them boys be, Hap," said Peaches, stepping out of shadow. "Jesus gathers even fancy boys to him. I don't care what that Brother Felcher over to Dry Prong says. He cain't know God's heart for sure. Ain't that right, Dopey Dwindle?"

Dopey cough-barked a fervent amen.

Back inside the RV, we folded down the longer couch for you, and I lay with you awhile. Your breath smelled like a high school chemistry lab.

Bonnie woke us in the morning, popping a can of Tab, fumbling through the locker over the microwave for a coffee pot. "I know I have one somewhere," she muttered. Suddenly she froze, glancing out the window. Bonnie opened the door to head Peaches off before she could knock.

"Brung you over some bran muffins," Peaches said. "They not raised up like they usually is, maybe 'cause of the altitude, but Hap says they's tasty."

"Thanks," said Bonnie, cracking open the screen door. "We're not awake yet."

"It looks as if Dopey Dwindle might have had something to do with making those muffins," you said.

Bonnie glanced down at the paper plate in her hand, at the flat brown cakes, then flicked them into the trash can.

III

Like you, Death Valley poised between vitality and depletion. I had never seen so clearly the fulcrum between life and death that everyone dances on, except now by your side. You and I arced together into a spiral of gain and forfeiture.

We drove west a ways to Ubehebe Crater, volcano-blasted out eons ago. Bonnie trudged to the rim, squinted down the 600-foot walls ringed in bands of orange and schist gray, lit a cigarette, coughed: "I suppose you two intend to hike the rim trail? Be back before dark. There's coyotes out there."

Our shadows stretched far over the desert or, as we rounded the rim, streaked deep into the crater, edgy projections spanning space and time notched in the crater's dimming striations.

Once I saw a Victorian seascape painting which I have never forgotten: several figures walk a sandy spit dwarfed by the sea before them. A woman looks directly out, towered over by a cliff layered with geological strata suggestive of earth shift and incessant slow change. The bands in the cliff are studded with fossils. The human figures seem disoriented: the woman's frown registers a new understanding that the cozy, providential world of her ancestors is instead schemed in chance and indifference. She gathers her skirts against a bitter sea, bones backing her in the cliff like a rigid curtain. She and her companions are displaced ciphers in the vastness of meaningless natural processes.

I put my arm around your waist. Violet shadows crept toward us, lapping up the silvery chaparral. The purple mountains to the west were edged in copper. I had never felt more tied to this earth than then, as much a part of it as the wildflowers and the mountains around me. This was home, almost certainly the only one I would ever know.

Do all lovers feel this grounding? Did you feel it, suspended with me on that shining path while a lilac-gray darkness sifted around us like dust? Learning to love was learning something new about how to be in the world. This growing bond between us spun out connecting filaments that brought all things inside and outside of me into coherence.

IV

In the morning, we set out for the sand dunes just outside of Stovepipe Wells. I wanted to see them while the sun shone slant. We rose early, postponed breakfast, Bonnie grumbling like a badger roused several weeks short of spring.

"You know I don't walk, Lu," she snapped when I asked her to join us. She steered the RV off Highway 190, tires crunching on the gravel shoulder. She popped a can of Tab and reached absently for a cigarette, already into her western.

We climbed, then half-slid down dune haunches. All we could see was sky and an endless angular succession of sun-burnt sand and lavender shadow. I moved my hand down your back to feel its planes, how it angled past your narrow hips to your indented flanks. Body and landscape prompted again the startling realization: love had led me out of myself into connection with another and then into larger spheres—comet tracks, craters, shifting dunes. The world became home in ways it never had been before.

"Uh-oh, look," you pointed. Away off in the distance we saw two RVs, rectangular clones dazzling on the horizon, the first one's broad windshield an S.O.S. semaphore in the sunlight. Our RV looked as if it had whelped.

"We'd better go and rescue Bonnie," I said.

She was sitting with the Dwindles in a cozy threesome of lawn chairs on the shady side of their rig.

"Peaches is a life master at bridge!" exclaimed Bonnie as we rushed up to relieve her. "We've been talking duplicate and Hoyle and new bidding strategy and who knows what all. She's headed to Vegas to play in a tournament. I'm going to register for it too."

"You boys had fun?" asked Hap, sunning thin legs angry with red splotches of eczema.

"Revelatory," I said. "Transfigurative."

"Ya'll been reading a dictionary up them dunes?" asked Hap.

We heard a rapping like upholstery needles raking over glass.

"Look!" said Peaches. "Dopey Dwindle's getting ready to put on his little show."

Dopey wobbled at the side window of the RV, mincing on the back of the couch under it. He glanced rapidly around to see that he had our attention, then dropped from sight.

"Wait," said Peaches.

Dopey popped up again. He cocked his head sharply to the left and froze. From his grizzled snout and thin black lips looped fluffy dust woozies, apparently gathered from some sweep-up pile. His eye darted sideways, saw we were laughing, darted back, froze in place. Suddenly he sneezed violently, sending the dust woozies floating around him like the ghosts of little gray puppies. He glanced quickly at his audience and dropped from view.

"Wait," said Peaches.

Dopey popped up again, a red ball clamped between his jaws, his eyes bulging. He ratatatated his toenails on the window like a drum roll, reared back, and coughed the ball onto the glass. He caught it on the rebound. He whined a thin violin tune in C-sharp for a moment, reared back, and expelled the ball again. It ricocheted with such force this time that it knocked him for a loop, rat tail over hairless haunches. Dopey immediately surfaced, ball clamped firmly in his jaws. He scanned the audience below with distended eyes, then ducked the slobbered ball on the sofa back, holding it there with one paw. He licked his chops and yawned.

We broke into applause.

"Learned that all by hisself," grinned Hap. "Dog's smart as me!"

"Un-hunh," said Bonnie. "Now about this bridge tournament, Peaches."

V

Bonnie was the most sedentary human being I have ever met. She was content to let the world approach her while she sat waiting for it, a wary eye alert to its tricks. But she humored you and me, stopping the RV before lunch so that we could take one more hike, far beneath the hanging rocks of Golden Canyon ending at the Red Cathedral.

We were alone on the trail. All we could see in any direction were primary colors at their most saturated. Rocks coded the canyon in sun-dipped canary. The sky above was a glazed blue emptiness, impermeable as porcelain. The Red Cathedral ended the canyon in eroded towers of frozen blood. All around us were chthonic forces unleashed, then restrained: arrested cataclysm.

I snapped a photograph of you in the shadow of a rock niche in the red cathedral wall. You lowered yourself slowly and sat on the rock step, hunched forward.

"Tired?" I asked.

"Maybe a little," you said.

On the way back, we stopped in a remaining square of sunlight. You leaned against the yellow wall, tilted your head back, the sun full on you.

"More than tired?" I fretted.

"Let's just rest a moment."

Again AIDS intruded on us: this was a trek between contraction and expansion. You looked ill and drawn; I was opening up to the world you seemed then on the verge of retreating from.

We had been gone almost two hours. When we returned to the rig, you napped, and I walked, alone, along a dirt road through white-crusted borate fields below leaden hills. No sound broke the tinny silence. "This is what I will have if you leave me!" The words erupted unbidden, my unconscious apparently anticipating your absence.

At the Badwater Basin you wanted to view the chemical desert, a drainage so saturated with salts that nothing could live there, not bacteria, not even viruses, a completely antibiotic zone bordering the point of lowest elevation in the United States (-282 feet).

The Dwindles had arrived just before we had. Peaches was trying to coax Dopey out of the rig with a doggy treat shaped like a cartoon bone, but he was not budging. He would crane his neck out to sniff the treat, do a little tap dance with his front feet, wriggle until he toppled over.

"It's a devil place is why he won't go out," said Hap. "Just leave him be."

As Peaches closed the rig door, we could hear Dopey's high whining.

"Critter's half bat," croaked Hap.

The water looked to be setting into stone. You stepped out on what seemed solid and broke through, water seeping up over the top of your shoe. Within minutes it rimed over, as if you were skeletonizing before our eyes.

"Let's leave this awful place," I said, pouring my drinking water over your shoe. "We need to get to Zabriskie Point in time to watch the sun set."

We followed the Dwindles to their rig.

"I'll see you in Vegas," said Bonnie to Peaches. "Let's play a round of bridge, if you can fit me in."

"Bye, Dopey," I said as Peaches opened the rig door. Dopey wriggled until he fell over, raised a leg and licked his privates with an obscene rose-petal tongue, scrambled up, cough-barked a couple of times.

VI

We arrived at Zabriskie Point right before sundown. The Point was crowded, but we found a place to stand at the rock-rim. A complete valley palette of colors ripened in the fading light.

You perched on a perimeter rock and held out your hand, your fingers alight as if gloved in gold leaf. You passed your hand slowly above the glowing sand. Then you laid your hand flat on the earth and rested it, like Siddhartha did on calling the earth to witness his enlightenment.

"The light is so heavy I thought I might be able to feel it," you said.

The sun descended behind a ridge, throwing a rinsed green glow, tremulous and clear, that soon dimmed to a purple gray. Suddenly, a splotch of coppery light blurred above the horizon.

People pointed.

"What's that?" asked Bonnie.

"The comet Hale-Bopp," I said. "It's a blessing over our beginning."

On our last night in Death Valley we made reservations at the Furnace Creek Inn for dinner. We walked through the dark palm gardens, wind rattling glassy fronds high above us. The Funeral Mountains cut a jagged black gash across a silver-studded sky.

At dinner, we sat at a white table by the windows looking out over the salt flats far below us. The moon had risen, a lopsided urn spilling silver. The borates on the flats glittered like hoarfrost. My back was to the dining room, across the table from you, Bonnie to my right.

Suddenly I saw soaring, open-mouthed columns twirling across the salt flats far below, dipping in slow white waltzes, three or four of them framing you.

"What are they?" I asked, motioning.

You turned around.

Bonnie craned sideways to see.

"Dust devils," said a hovering waiter in black and white, holding a silver water carafe. "The desert winds have kicked them up."

The macabre dancers swayed and bowed and drifted over the moonlit borate plain. We watched those tall writhings of ash through the windows, my hand slipping over your hand across the table.

GARDENS

I

Spring is early and long and languorous in Sacramento. It steals a peep through January fog and then retreats. Its first revisions are tentative: a trace of pale blossoms along the branches of a wild plum.

In late January, Spring begins to think the color green too long out of fashion. It tints the tips of the elderberry canes a celadon so cautious that one loses it if one looks directly at it. Then one morning in February, the grasses, battered low by winter rains and left for dead, announce a rinsed green revival. Later, the Bradford pears spume and sputter, their white florets sperm-scented.

In March, Spring grows as self-assured as a girl playing her second piano recital. The mourning doves return, flickering silver-gray. Pale sunlight haloes in grasses prinked with orange poppies and blue lupines.

By April, Spring is tomboy-cocky. The honey-locusts hang out their sweet white clusters, as delicate as Meissen porcelain. Then the pink jasmine elbows up my garden fence and busts into full bloom with a scent so intense that it clobbers the heart.

I loved the rhythms of our bodies on a fragrant April morning, how we moved in slow cadence, how my tongue wound a path to your nipples, anticipating a greater treasure, accumulating interest. That April morning the outside bedroom door ajar and sunlight, spiked with birdsong, pouring in, I crossed into a dazzling garden where nothing is said with words before one returns to a rumpled

90

sheet and the sound of our breathing like gusts through blooming laurel, a wedge of sunlight drizzling your bare calf.

We dressed and drove to my house. Winter storms had loosened the brads on the grape arbor over the second-floor veranda. You stood on a ladder to secure the trailing vines to the arbor frame. While you worked, I came over to lip the scar on your bare knee.

You laughed and wriggled your leg as if shooing a persistent fly. "You are such a pervert," you said.

"And what kind of person hangs out with perverts?" I asked.

"A therapist," you said. "I'm here to help you."

Then we tackled the garden fountain, clearing out dead leaves and winter muck. With the fountain chuckling in new water, I tilled the garden and planted seeds. Planting a spring garden is like beginning a love affair—that same eagerness to see what, if anything, will thrive.

II

The next day, a Sunday, I drove to Corey's to deliver his meds from the Foundation and to spell Beau, Corey's home-health-care aide. I had been assigned to Corey a month after Sean gargled to his end with two volunteers from the Foundation monitoring his morphine drip.

Corey was end-stage. For years I had seen him at monthly Foundation potlucks. He had been buoyant as a fishing bob through a school of hungry sharks: PCP, thrush, cytomegalovirus. Now he was being yanked under by kidney disease, hepatitis C, and thrombocytopenic purpera, where his body no longer produced sufficient platelets to allow clotting. Large purple continents mapped his arms and torso.

Corey's landlord had installed burglar bars over the windows of his ground-floor apartment after a third break-in. The tenant upstairs, a heavy man on disability and methadone, paced back and forth, footfalls thudding down all day and a good part of the night, always out of synch with the base from the heavy metal rock he played incessantly.

The apartment was sweltering. Always cold now, Corey wore an athletic tooth-guard to help prevent his chills from shattering his teeth. Light hurt his eyes, so one red light bulb lit the bedroom like a photo lab. Glinting in a corner was a tinsel palm tree left over from his days as a travel agent. He could not stand to be touched, except very lightly, so Beau had not bathed him for several days.

"Who's he?" croaked Corey when I entered the bedroom. "Tell him to go away. I don't want him here." Corey had to turn his head at an odd angle to look at me through the thin edge of peripheral vision remaining to him. He resembled a petulant child afraid to face what had emerged from under the bed.

"It's Lu, Corey," said Beau. "You know Lu. Why do you want him to go away?"

A long pause. . . .

"Because he's going to cry. I don't want anyone to cry."

"I'll try my best not to cry, Corey." I laid my hand on the bump in the blanket where his hands were. "Let me just sit here with you for a while."

Corey's head sank back on his pillow. Soon he was asleep, murmuring occasionally to Chaz, the cockatoo he had had to give up several months before.

Corey stirred when the apartment door opened on Beau's return, but he did not awaken.

"Beau's back, Corey. I'm going to go now."

Corey woke with a start and turned his head sideways to look up at me. He extended his hand from under the covers. "I'm going to go now too. There's no use in this anymore, Lu."

I nodded and rested the back of my hand lightly on his cheek for a moment.

Outside, a breeze wafted through a flowering magnolia to the side of the door. Under it was the little garden Corey and I had planted several months before. He had admired some geraniums in my yard, a maroon blossom veined in pale pink. I had rooted some cuttings for him, but they were struggling in the shade. Cigarette butts now littered the plot, tossed down by the tenant upstairs.

Two hours after I left, Corey's caseworker from the Foundation called. Corey had died moments after his brother had arrived from Reno. His brother had reported that some cash, a gold chain, and Corey's high-school graduation ring were missing. He was changing the locks. He wanted to know what to do with the meds I had delivered that morning.

III

After I got the call, I phoned you: "Okay if I come over early?" The rank odor of Corey's apartment had stayed with me, even after I had gotten home.

93

"Corey's gone?"

"Yes," I said, "shortly after I left him."

"The garden party will do us good."

People drifted in and out of Mary T. and Robert's house, up and down the rows of roses. We sat under a pergola bending under a pink cascade of climbing Cecile Brunners, listening to a mockingbird scaling his repertoire and to the muffled voices wafting to us down the rose paths.

The afternoon was fresh, a soft breeze stirring the lilacs and the new clouds drifting directionless in the upper air. I sat close to you. Swerves and veerings of light larked over us, rose tints, lances and penumbras, light cavorting like water in a fountain. If heaven be a regained garden, I prayed, do not let it be static and breathless. Let there be ripple and caper and blow and a wild energy that drives the tulips and a zest that forces the lilies. Or let us give up heaven altogether and remain here, in this terrestrial garden, a part of all this forever.

You reached up for a swag knotted with roses and pricked your finger, a tiny ruby forming on its tip.

I offered you my handkerchief.

"We'd better not," you said. No one was more cautious about spreading HIV than you, even when the precaution was unnecessary.

You stood. We wound down the paths to see guests palming plates and sipping wine and Mary T. holding forth and Robert pointing out to Senator Ortiz the new green ceramic cat crouching on the lip of a square pool arcing water from its mouth in a silvery splash.

IV

I have a lingering memory of an April morning almost exactly one year after Mary T. and Robert's garden party. I brought the cushions out of the garage for the first time that year and laid them on the teakwood chaise for you. A breeze capered through the redwoods, fretting you in light and shade. I planted two new rose bushes I had bought for you. You watched me, the newspapers still rolled tightly and resting against your robed thigh.

It was the day after Mary T. and Robert's garden party that year. You were too sick to attend, though you had urged me to go. I had not the heart to go without you.

"If you can't come to the roses," Mary hollered when I answered the sunset knock at the door last evening, "the roses will come to you." She handed me a bouquet.

"Can't stay," Robert had said, extending a plate of cookies. "Someone backed into my delphinium bed and broke several canes. It's a hopeless triage, but I have to try to stake them up."

I lugged several flats of purple impatiens out of your garage, darker than the lavender ones you usually planted.

"Are you very disappointed?" I asked. "This is the lightest shade I could find."

"They're beautiful," you said.

You were as translucent as bone porcelain in that pale sunlight. I laid each one of those impatiens sprigs in a purple mantle bordering the path and the redwood trees you had planted years before. The gloom under the redwoods glimmered with star jasmine.

"Smell this," I said, offering you a star. "The fuchsias are budding too. They'll soon be mincing around in their puce pantaloons, the gay little things."

You took the jasmine star and raised it to your nostrils. You closed your eyes and inhaled deeply. You danced the star lightly over your lips, your eyes still closed.

"I am so very happy!" I whispered.

You opened your eyes wide and smiled at me with delight, the coefficient of Spring itself and all its gardens.

RHODODENDRONS

I

To me, rhododendrons were simply azaleas with attitude. I grew up with azaleas: in Louisiana, they are scattered about every yard, beautiful in cultivated massings but too often untended. Then they spread out white, pink, or mournful purple bundles like ragged clothes drying on bushes in the hen-pecked yards of sharecropper shotgun houses.

You had read in the San Francisco <u>Chronicle</u> that the rhododendrons in Golden Gate Park were offering the most spectacular display in years.

"Want to go?" you asked.

Ummm, okay," I hesitated. "We can spend the day in the de Young Museum, maybe catch the Pops at the band shell. What say I bring a picnic?"

We woke on Sunday morning to a wetness dumping itself like a damp cat into the bedroom through the open door to the garden. I leaned on the doorjamb looking out at sparrows hunkered on low branches, dribbling depressed chirps and ruffling the wet off, all nest building suspended. A crow stalked the gloom under the redwoods like a priest burdened by the sins confessed the day before.

"It'll clear," you assured me from the bed, your eyes still closed.

"Doesn't matter," I said. "We could spend the whole day in the de Young. We can have our picnic under the pergola."

97

"But you have to see the rhodies against a clear sky," you said. "Rhodies have to be backlit."

"Rhodies? You're a garden-club lady on intimate terms with all her flower friends?"

"Maybe," you said, "but I'm a garden-club lady with wayward tastes, and now it's time to plant the tuber. Why don't you come back to bed."

I loved having drowsy sex in the morning: sex in slow motion, the driving vigor of the night's urgency having spent itself. It was like eating when one is no longer hungry, but the food laid before one is bountiful and luscious. It was like loving you under water, drifting in undulations, touch like calm ripples. The bodies of true lovers piece together in a connection unavailable to those enjoying the enormous but fickle pleasures of one-night stands.

Our coming was a slow gathering rather than the whistling upheaval of the night before. But always, always I feared: can the virus coiled in the cum you spilled on me enter through a tiny cut in my hand? a hangnail? A scratch I do not know about? And this drove me out of the tossed pillows to wash right away.

In the shower, you angled me so that my back was to you. "The rhodies are waiting for us," you whispered.

II

You drove. Across the green bay, San Francisco's bridges and spires floated against a sky the blue of parrot feathers.

We parked close to the Spreckels Bandshell and laid out the picnic: a slab of pate', a wedge of blue cheese, slices of olive bread, and early pears green as duck eggs.

You poured only a half glass of dry rose' for yourself: wine burned your throat lately. You had a post-nasal drip, you surmised, that would not go away. It hurt whenever you swallowed.

"You've thought of every detail, as usual," you said. "Every color and shape and taste."

"Turn a blind eye to life and we slip through it too fast."

"Don't you ever feel weary? Burdened by it all?" you asked. "I sometimes worry about what may be coming."

"I used to be afraid a lot—of getting on a plane, of being in a car wreck, you name it," I said, leery of cliches. "But I don't face life alone anymore. Neither do you. I can't imagine my life without you."

You looked about to say something but thought better of it.

At the de Young, we saw a loan exhibit of Monet's last canvases produced during his final retreat to Giverny, his eyes failing him. The water lilies in his garden ponds were mere paint blobs, the eyebrow bridge a maroon smear of memory and blurred sight. Ugly and yet moving, they opened windows into loss, the land we all steadily approach.

"Let's exit through Greek antiquities," you suggested, scanning the map in the museum brochure.

We had the sculpture corridors to ourselves. Not even a guard was in sight. White gods and goddesses gestured in dim halls. A plaster cast of Apollo arrested us. Its chest and shoulders were yours, but its abdomen was broader. Its raised arms, broken off at the wrists, were bent at the elbows. I saw you again in this morning's bed, your arms thrown back.

"What I love about these sculptures," I said, "is that the Greeks combined physical beauty with moral virtue. Their Christian successors insist on mortifying the body to perfect the soul."

"We gay men seem to prize the body above all things. We can't seem to forgive each other when our bodies give way," you added. "But then I won't have to worry about any of that."

"I am the quintessential pagan," I said. "I adore you, body and soul."

"I don't want to be adored," you said, hurrying me forward with one hand on my shoulder.

III

The exit lay just through the last Greek corridor. We came to a broken stone bracketed to a wall. A man in a wheelchair sat in front of it. He appeared to be dozing, head fallen forward over his chest in that sad, uncomfortable way of old people left in wheelchairs parked along the urine-odorous halls of nursing homes.

As we approached, he roused himself. I will never get used to it, I thought, these youths wasted into old men as if by a fairy tale curse, these withered boys balding from toxic meds, faces a splotchy brown-purple, and eyes in which fever and fatigue dulled but failed to blot out completely youth's keen flash.

He had dropped a medicine vial beside his chair. I picked it up and handed it to him.

"Cliff's gone for water," he said.

"Perhaps I should roll you to a fountain?" I answered. "I'm not sure he'll be allowed to bring water to you in the galleries."

"I'd better wait so Cliff will know where I am."

The broken stone bracket before us was a funerary stele incised with two male figures. The first stood in three-quarter high relief, his back to the viewer. His right hand reached towards the other figure standing in shallow bas-relief across a blank divide. This second figure, naked, seemed to be receding into the stone. He gazed at the first figure with a serene melancholy. One arm fell by his side; the other was raised, a valedictory gesture extending over the divide, their fingers not quite touching.

"They were lovers," the man in the wheelchair said.

"How do you know?" I asked, scanning the museum label.

"Look at them. Look at their ages, their gestures."

"Lovers, then," I said.

"I need to sit for a while," you said. "And I have pills to take."

IV

"I had no idea!" I breathed as I followed you into the first grove. The purple rhododendron bracts towered at least twenty feet above us. Amethyst tinctured the thin light. Your lips looked like slices of ripe plum.

The purple rhododendron grove faded into a pink room through a violet rosy gradation. Dawn clouds spumed above us. The pistil of each pink floret arced out like a scarlet wire; each stamen was beaded in a vermilion testicle. The throats of the florets were speckled with an orange measling.

"See?" you said.

"Let's live together in these rosy towers forever!"

"The sun's setting," you frowned.

"Let it," I said. "We'll love these rooms in moonlight."

"No," you said. "Soon we'll have to leave."

We stumbled a short turning further into a white chamber loftier than any we had yet entered, a hollowed pearl. Each white blossom reeled out a light, laughing furl of teasing song, intuited rather than heard. I took you in my arms. You started, looked quickly around, then relaxed. A shadow pooled in the recess of your cheek. Neither of us said a word.

The light shifted: the white rhododendrons instantly distilled a silvery lavender—the single perfect moment in this perfect day.

AXILLA

Where the play's climax, lushly scripted, often had its prologue.

Where I mined for golden pleasure, squandering it on you even as I gleaned it.

Where, like a snail from copper, my tongue recoiled from the astringency of your antiperspirant, the bitter relish of uncured olives, unripe persimmons, the yellowing ends of mid-September cucumbers left too long on their drying vines.

Where the fine long hair whirled in loose orbs, the vortices of my desire.

Where two pale valleys inclined, redolent of wheat and the tartness of the grape, ground of the erotic sacrament I took on my tongue.

Where, with your arms raised, you were my giving-up, most mine, my thrall, I your servant holding my emancipation fee simple.

Where I found my place reserved, exclusive possession, my staked claim, eminent domain.

Where, saddled by my tongue, you bucked in pleasure's reins.

Where the way to your bronze nipples and opened lips traced a slick, silver trail.

Where my tongue burrowed, like a squirrel returning in autumn dusk to its hidden granary in a red maple quoin, secure from fox and owl.

Where I construed in those downed declensions the grammar of my need.

Where I returned to nest after my singing flight along the branches of your body.

Where my tongue sought early one morning to savor you and stumbled instead on a bulging lymph node, tender, treacherous, hard as a stone, raising for us the first high slope of your illness.

This is my paean to your armpit.

MAY DAY

Your doctor assured you that patients with HIV frequently presented with lymphadenopathy or swollen lymph nodes. Nothing to worry about. They would do tests.

But that was not what worried us, what pained you. You began to pick at your food, to swallow hesitantly, grimacing. Then you began to eat very little. Your throat hurt all the time, you said. The doctor said allergies. You took Claritin. Tonsillitis, the doctor said when antihistamines did not help. You took antibiotics. Maybe thrush? More antibiotics.

You paced the house at night in pain, silently, or you left our bed to lie on the couch in the family room. I would hear from bed the murmur of the television with its 3:00 A. M. carnival of freaks, charlatans, televangelists, its tired re-runs of corny sit-coms and polyester detective shows. I would walk out into the family room, blue as an aquarium in the television glare, to see you lying under a blanket, your eyes white porcelain.

"Go back to bed," you would urge gently. "I'm just a little restless. I'll sleep out here for a while."

I carried back to bed the image of you shrunken under a brown blanket, emblem of vulnerability and pain.

I woke one morning and saw it, just under your right jaw.

"This is no tonsillitis or throat infection, Dore, and no swollen lymph node," I said in alarm, running a finger lightly over the swelling. "This is nothing antibiotics can help."

"They've scheduled a biopsy for a week from today," you said quietly. "They think it may be internal Kaposi's sarcoma on the bronchi or maybe a tumor. I was going to tell you."

Our dread met a distraction: my parents and my sister Felice arrived for a visit planned months before. They were eager to meet you. Your throat hurt all the time now. You could manage only a few tentative bites at meals.

At Lake Tahoe we had dinner at the buffet on the top floor of Harrah's, more for the view than for the food. You positioned a thin slice of rare prime rib and a jot of mashed potatoes on your plate, ate nothing. My father glanced at the server bearing your uneaten plate away, glanced at me, eyebrows raised.

My family returned to Louisiana without knowing of your illness. I peered helplessly into your throat every day with a flashlight at a glistening red wound scalloped in black from the biopsy. Your weight had begun to drop alarmingly.

It was a late Friday afternoon, the last of May, hot, after your day at work. Earlier in the afternoon, I had attended a memorial service, my second that week. I had sat dry-eyed with other stunned witnesses from the AIDS Foundation. For the second time that week, a recording of Louis Armstrong's version of "It's a Wonderful World" ended the service.

"What do you know?" I asked, cautious.

"It's non-Hodgkin lymphoma," you said blithely.

"Not Kaposi's?"

"No."

"Is it worse than Kaposi's?"

"Don't know," you said. "I have to go through chemo. I'm in an early stage, which I'm told is good. It's not in the nervous system. It should respond well to treatment. The doctor is optimistic. I see an oncologist Monday." You smiled brightly.

"Sounds like this is more treatable than Kaposi's?

"Sounds like it."

I started rinsing lettuce for a salad. The phone rang. It was your sister Bonnie calling from Seattle. She wanted to know. You told her the biopsy results with exactly the same buoyant tone you used with me, the exact words, the bright smile. Then your voice broke.

"I know that," you strangled, then handed the phone to me without another word to Bonnie.

"What's for supper?" Bonnie asked.

"Salad," I said, wrestling with the word, trying to breathe. "Baked chicken, potato," I edged out, the words thick.

Bonnie ignored the sodden tone. "What are your plans?" she asked. "For tonight."

"Television. We're staying in," I got out. You came up behind me, put your arms around me, your cheek against the side of my head.

"Talk to you soon," Bonnie said brightly, the Tanner way.

"I <u>hate</u> that," you hissed when I hung up.

"What?" I asked. "What did she say?"

"She said she would always be there for me, that anything I needed. . . if ever the time came. . . . I knew that already. I hate that talk."

I willed tears not to well over. I would not give them up.

"Me too," I said.

CENTERING

In early June, we flew to Seattle for a weekend holiday with Bonnie before you started chemotherapy. At Pike Street Market, I backed up to take a photograph of you posed in an aisle between vendor displays. To your left was a fishmonger's stall. Dungeness crabs tatted their blue legs into loose webs inside a dripping wood-slat box. A grit-crusted hummock of oysters squatted next to them like ill-tempered toads. A shadowy green tank cloistered a coven of lobsters.

The cases to your right held a truck farmer's produce. Nectarines nestled in a tray next to white peaches, their furred butt-clefts bottoms up. Strawberries oozed like dislodged hearts, dark seeds dinting them with little sorrows. A bay of kiwis, resembling mossed brook stones, rounded the transition to the vegetables.

Carrots lay crossed like pick-up-sticks. Spires of green broccoflower rose like the towers of Mormon temples. Bell peppers jostled each other, glossed in green chrome. Bunches of scallions lay rigid, disapproving of an invasive clown-tumble of radishes.

Here you are, grounded in that bounty, frowning into the camera, put out at the delay as I angled the camera this way and that to catch you best. All things surround you, catalyst of color and contour. Here you are in this photograph in my hand all these years later, still demurring, still centering my vision.

PART III: THE CARDS IN THE BOX

Foreseeing the possibility of life without
Possibility of joy, let him give it up.
--Wendell Berry, "Three Elegiac Poems"

CLINIC

I

We pulled up under the oncology clinic porte-cochere on a June morning still cool from the evening's delta breezes. Parking attendants in khaki shorts and white polo shirts intercepted every arriving vehicle. They looked like tennis pros swarming a country club rather than ushers for the ill. One of them scanned me quickly, flashed a glance your way, looked back at me. "Do you need help, sir?" he asked me. You laughed. "I think we can both manage," I replied.

The full waiting room in the chemo unit represented a diorama of the arbitrary, fate handing out illnesses carelessly. A woman in tailored culottes and a hard wig flicked through a magazine and glanced repeatedly at her wristwatch. A blue bruise spread over the valley below her biceps. Across from her drooped a tiny man blinking liquid eyes, his cough like the splat of blood-soaked cotton dropped on linoleum. "Gramma," moaned a toddler collapsed on the flat breast of an alert old lady. The toddler was bald and beak-mouthed like a tortoise. "I know, honey. We're going home soon," the old lady whispered.

"Look, it's Hugh!" I whispered, nudging you.

Hugh had seen us. He motioned us over.

"It's Jeff," he said, "not me. He's got Hodgkin's lymphoma, a bad kind, and cancer of the jaw. He didn't want anyone to know yet."

Hugh put his head down. "He should be nearly done with today's chemo. He didn't want me there."

You sat down next to him and laid a hand on his knee. "I'm here for something similar," you said.

"Oh no," Hugh looked up, his eyes glistening.

"My case doesn't look so bad,"

"Will this ever STOP?" Hugh cried. "I don't think I can take much more."

A nurse came out scanning your chart.

"Do you want to go in alone?" I asked.

"You come," you said.

The nurse ushered us into a small room where you sat on the examining table, crackling the parchment-paper drawn down over it, your legs dangling. The walls were completely bare.

"Who is this harder on, do you think? Hugh or Jeff?

"I'd say Jeff," I said.

"I'm not so sure," you replied. "This may be rough on both of us."

We were silent for a moment.

Then: "Dr. Choy. Do you know what her first name is?" you asked.

I shrugged.

"Pansy. Pansy Choy. I looked her up on the clinic website. She had a bio: parents Chinese immigrants from Hong Kong. She's got two sisters: Violet and Daisy. All three Stanford Medical."

"A medical nosegay!" I laughed.

Dr. Choy opened the door. She flipped the pages of your chart. The essence of unflappability, she soothed one to look at her.

"I'm certain the lymphoma diagnosis was a blow," she said, "but the good news is that you are in stage one of the disease, which means there's no involvement beyond the original tumor. This type of immunodeficient Burkitt's lymphoma responds well to chemotherapy. Here are two recent articles I've copied for you advocating lower doses of chemo for patients with early disease progression. If you agree, we'll go this route, especially in light of your HIV status. That should keep any side effects minimal. Questions?"

"I've tried to read everything I can on the lymphoma websites. There's a lot out there," you said. "Apparently this kind of lymphoma is not uncommon in AIDS patients given large doses of AZT for a length of time?"

"That's right. We're seeing a lot of this type of non-Hodgkin lymphoma. But I think you'll see rapid results on the tumor, even as pronounced as this one is." She palpated the tumor. "Big as a tulip bulb."

I laughed. Dr. Choy glanced curiously at me, then away.

"Next stop is the chemo station," she said.

Dr. Choy's stride was more flow than walk, matching her efficient containment. She glided us into a room floored in oak and flooded by light from floor-to-ceiling glass bays, each centered by two lounge chairs. The tiny man with liquid eyes was being digested by one of the chairs; it sucked him into its middle like a starfish ingesting a scallop. Tubes connected him to a yellow solution in a glistening plastic bag like the flayed carcass of a fat dachshund.

Dr. Choy introduced us to a nurse named Kali, a middle-aged woman with a bad ginger poodle-perm and large purple glasses. Glimpsed through her lenses, her temples looked indented on each side, as if her head had been squeezed in a vise. She wore a v-necked smock scattered with green palm trees and hula girls. Huge pineapples floated about, threatening to crush anything beneath if gravity re-claimed them.

"Each session will last a little over an hour," Kali said. "Bring your favorite CDs or videos."

"Side effects?" I asked.

"We don't expect them to be significant," she said and beamed.

"See," you said to me. "He's always worrying over nothing."

"There could be some nausea on occasion, some fatigue, lowered red or elevated white blood counts," she continued, "but they should be minimal, if they occur at all."

"And this?" I laughed, grabbing a lock of the hair falling over your forehead.

"Oh, he'll lose that," said Kali.

Suddenly, without warning or knowing where they came from, I was gulping sobs. The nature of the ordeal became real to us at that moment.

Kali interjected quietly: "Your prognosis is excellent, Dore, and your hair will grow back."

Once outside, the Sacramento sun pressed a hot hand heavy on us.

"I need a haircut," you said.

You had just had your hair styled and highlighted—expensively, perfectly.

"If I have to lose it, I don't want it this long when it falls out."

"Haircut?" a stylist asked me as we entered a SuperCuts down the street. Her thin hair was pulled up so tightly into a topknot that she looked like a garlic bulb.

"Yes," I said, "and one for him too."

She scanned your hair, puzzled, uncertain.

"Shorter," you said. "Me first."

The stylist picked up a scissors and comb and then hesitated. "How short?"

"I want a crew cut," you said. "Use clippers."

"Are you sure?" she asked.

"How about a quarter inch all around?"

"You'll see scalp for at least three weeks," she said.

"I wish it were for only that long," you said. "Cut away."

The sift of your hair soon littered the floor. You looked like a bewildered army recruit, away from home for the first time, eyes stretched rounder, mouth wider, Adam's apple knobbier.

When she finished, you brisked your hand back and forth over your head. Cut stubble flew around like ecstatic midges.

I rubbed my hand over your scalp. "Feels like a toilet bowl brush."

"Cruel thing," you said.

"You next? How do you want it?" asked the stylist.

"Exactly the same," I said.

"No you don't," you protested. "This is *my* summer look. Get your own."

"I'll make the sides similar," whispered the stylist.

"One last errand before we go home," you said, the two of us, newly lopped, blinking in the sun. "Let's go to Macy's."

"Ooooh, shopping!"

"I want to buy a broad-brimmed straw hat. . . ."

". . . . like old geezers wear in the Sacramento sun?"

"Not helpful," you said. "Chemo makes you sun-sensitive. I'll broil without hair."

Before shopping, we had to visit the men's room in the Macy's downtown. All the stall doors were closed. On our entrance, heads popped up to peer over the toilet enclosures at us, one after another in the row.

"Husbands!" I fussed. "Wives waiting and lawns to mow in Orangevale and Citrus Heights and Carmichael. Oh, not gay, of course. Just after a little of what their wives won't give them. They'll condemn us in their fundy churches, these Sunday-school sneaks!"

You selected a broad-brimmed Panama with a khaki hatband centered by a leather buckle. You shot a wistful look in a mirror.

"Stand still," I ordered. I tilted the hat at an angle. You looked like a Miami gangster. I righted the hat: you looked like a codger setting out to play poker and eat free spaghetti at the American Legion hall. I tipped the hat back. You looked like everyone's Uncle Charlie, thumbs in suspenders, arriving in time for aw-shucks Sunday pot roast. I tipped the hat forward. You came into focus. But you never saw this as the right way to wear it. You clapped the hat on any old way. Over time, I stopped noticing the many personas the hat disguised you with.

You nibbled at a salad for supper. Your weight continued to drop. I tried to bribe you to drink a can of high-calorie nutritional supplement I had bought without consulting you. You were adamant in rejecting it, the first of many stubborn tussles with me over your food.

"You'll sleep with me whether I drink it or not," you laughed. "That bribe won't work."

You read the paper, propped up by pillows. I dozed, awakened by the click of the lamp. We were soon naked in a wedge of moonlight, the delta breezes cool on our skin. I lipped the sculptural join at the saddle of your hips, our loving a humming tenderness; our coming, an echoing through the house. Afterwards, I seemed for a moment to look down on the body wreckage in the bed.

II

At the first administration of the chemotherapy, Kali sported a smock stamped in morning-glories and hummingbirds. Huge suns floated about, threatening to incinerate birds and blooms.

Kali sat you in one of the recliners; fussed with the adjustments; trotted out magazines and CDs like an airline attendant in first-class; pulled up a stainless-steel tray and a stand; zoomed in next to you on a wheeled chair.

You winced as she inserted the needle-intake into the back of your left hand and taped it in place. Into this port she buried another needle, a terminus for two thin plastic tubes. We heard a clicking as she adjusted the drip speed, a quiet whirring, and, with a pat and a murmur, she sped away.

The treatment area was empty in spite of the crowded waiting room. I moved to the recliner next to yours. We sat there like a long-married couple prepped for a dozy evening of television in our dual Barcaloungers.

A beeper sounded. Kali zoomed in on her wheeled chair, disconnected a bag, plumped another from the tray, spanked it like a newborn, asked how you were, zoomed away on her foot-propelled chair.

We heard another patient arrive.

"Jeff!" I said. "You'll need the chair. . . ."

"I'm not sure why anymore," Jeff said. "The chemo doesn't seem to be working. They've found new tumors. They wanted to cut part of my jaw away, but I refused that grotesque suggestion. They're trying a new regimen today, which means I have to start all over again. Ten weeks this time."

"Is Hugh with you?" I asked.

"No, I don't want him to come anymore. He gets too upset and gives the doctors a hard time. They're doing what they can."

"You two come over for dinner this Saturday," you said.

"We'll have to call you about that," Jeff said. "Right now the thought of eating anything makes me gag. But that'll be better in a few days, I hope."

They did not come for dinner that weekend. Or any other.

I monitored you that afternoon until you chafed at the attention, assuring me that rushing my hand to your forehead, hovering by the bathroom door, and sticking snacks in your face was not helping.

"Let me at 'em," you growled the next morning when I asked you how you felt. You went to work, came home as usual around 3:00, took your nap.

"I feel great," you said as we were undressing for bed two nights later.

You woke me early the next morning, nuzzling my ear. We took a shower together. I washed your hair. I pulled my hands down to rinse the suds off them. I could not see my palms for the matted felt. I held them up for you to see.

"I know," you said. "I saw it on the pillow this morning."

III

Sometimes I woke you by lightly fingering the swelling. You would start, blink, then throw your head back, baring your throat. The tumor had begun to shrink.

Not all your hair fell out. The whorls remaining hugged your skull like a fretwork cap. With so little hair, you seemed diminished, simultaneously old and boyish.

At your next chemo treatment, the pride of frat boy valets gleamed a white-toothed brilliance as they tore along on the balls of their feet, calves bulging like newel posts. "Help you, sir?" they asked you. No one needed to ponder which of us was a clinic patient now.

You bantered with the receptionists while you checked in, all middle-aged divorcees scouting out men whose wives were dying of breast cancer. The receptionists all liked you. You were handsome and tall, with a breezy insouciance rare in the frightened, rotten-feeling patients they dealt with all day. You were what the valet boys would grow into in twenty years, except you had a mind.

Dr. Choy of the floral sisterhood murmured barely audible inquiries as to how you were tolerating the chemo. She angled your head back gently and fingered the tumor lightly, as I had done that morning.

"Any other swellings?" she purled, moving her hands over your body.

"None I know of," you said, "except the lymph nodes."

"It's going well," she sighed. "As well as we had hoped. Your blood work looks fine. Ready for the next treatment?"

Kali greeted us in a smock imprinted with bulbous women in bikinis tossing huge beach balls all over it.

"What good results we've been getting about you, Dore." Kali scanned your chart, beaming like a parent reviewing a much-improved report card.

She hooked you up. This time the lounges were all occupied. In the chair next to you huddled a wizened nun in full habit, her face the color of the wimple framing it. She opened her eyes briefly when you sat down, studied Kali's smock a moment, closed them again.

"You seem so young to be here," she said, more to herself than to you. "Sometimes it's not clear to me that God always knows what He's doing."

"Sister Peter Claver?"

The old nun fluttered her eyes open.

"Used to be," she said. "Sister Mavis now. The sisters all went back to their birth names and I went along, though it's a dumb name for a nun. We've also got a Sister Debbie and a Sister Nikki. Kept the habit, though. I never could get the hang of panty hose. Did I teach you?"

"At St. Philomene's? Dore Tanner?"

"I remember your mother," the nun said. "All you kids looked alike."

"And this is my partner, Lu."

She looked me over and nodded. "Are you doing well, if that's not an absurd question in this place?"

"He's doing great!" said Kali, zooming in on her chair. "And you're done, Sister. Until next week. The porter's here to take you to the van."

122

"If I live until next week," the nun said. "I'm trying to persuade God He's gotten all He can get out of me by now, but He's apparently not having it."

"Sister!" chided Kali. "Now none of that!"

"You know, you don't have to come with me next time," you called over to me. "I mean, so far, this has been a piece of cake."

"I want to be with you when you hear the good news," I said.

Peter Pan took your car claim ticket and roared our car up from Neverland. A block or two away from the clinic, you pulled over and put the convertible top down, and we drove in a Sacramento summer sun just getting serious. You clamped your hat firmly to your head. Your ears bulged a bit to accommodate the brim.

"Where to for lunch?" I asked. "Let's celebrate!"

You swerved the car to the side of the street. You opened your door and leaned out, whisking your hat off. You vomited into the gutter. You righted yourself in your seat, propped your head on the rest. Then you leaned out and vomited again. You wiped your arm over your wet forehead, tears burning their way down your cheeks.

IV

So went the summer. You were working, though you took off on the chemo days. I had to skip a few of them, hired away to score high-school honor essays for a bit of summer money, a change of scene, an anonymous trick or two. We arranged a backup for chemo driving, but you never needed it. The lymphoma was all but in remission. You were three-quarters through the regimen.

School started for me. My teaching schedule allowed me to accompany you on the chemotherapy days. I would be on sabbatical leave the following term. We planned an early spring sojourn in Italy: hailing vaporetti in a wet, gray Venice together, then St. Peter's Square waving handkerchiefs during the pope's Easter blessing. We would return home well before the arrival of Rome's tourists and the onset of its summer heat.

Toward the end of September, we went for one of your last treatments. I drove us through streets under yellowing leaves not yet ready to call it quits. We pulled under the porte-cochere at the clinic. One of the Lost Boys opened your door. They all knew you by now.

"The good news first, Dore," Dr. Choy greeted you. "The lymphoma is in remission. We don't see any traces of it on the last scan. But your blood work's off, so we'll need to boost the count before we can complete the last treatments. This prescription is for that. Come back in two weeks for a new blood count. We'll conclude the treatments then."

We stopped off to tell Kali why you could not stay for your appointment. She had on a smock with little men in lederhosen, pinching sausages and folding pretzels. Enormous steins of beer zeppelined around them.

"Gearing up for Oktoberfest?" I asked. "Kali, what uniform shop do you buy these nurse get-ups from?"

"Buy?! I make them."

"Ohhh," I said. "That explains a lot."

It looked as if the same young man brought the car back who had driven it away, but we could not be certain.

"Let's go somewhere and be happy," I suggested.

"Didn't you hear Dr. Choy? We came all this way for nothing."

"I think I heard her say you were in remission. Fuck the blood cells. We'll give them a breather; then we'll buck them up."

You were reluctant.

"How about we drive out to Woodland?"

"What's there?"

"Well, the Costa del Sol, for one thing."

"Ptomaine Taqueria. Hepatitis Hacienda. I don't think so."

"Well, how about an afternoon in the antique shops on Main Street?"

"Dead people's stuff," you said.

How about the summer sales at the Emporium?"

"You and I both know those clothes are on brief reprieve before exile in Central America."

"Look," I said, "I would follow you to the ends of the earth. All I'm asking is for you to follow me the thirty miles to Woodland!"

On that aimless afternoon, a restrained joy seeped into our disappointment. All the world was working, and we were exempt, a fact I pointed out to you, which did not seem to comfort you much.

We walked the main street of downtown Woodland, a corridor of storefronts built late in the nineteenth century. If I cast my eyes at a certain slant, I would be back in Manhattan, Kansas. Only a few years before, I had walked a similar downtown Manhattan street alone. I had no idea then that I would soon migrate to California and love a mortal man with such joy and distress.

In an antique shop I bought you a teacup and saucer while you fiddled with a superannuated adding machine. I surprised you with the teacup later that evening as a gift to mark this day of remission. The saucer rim and the outside of the cup are the creamy green of duck eggs; the bottom of the cup bowl is painted with gold-brown leaves. I have that cup now. When I raise it to my lips and see the fall leaves through the yellow-green of my tea, I re-live that day and think of you with longing.

V

"We'll be late for your appointment," I said again.

"What does it matter?" you said, turning away from me.

The bouts of nausea were frequent over the last week.

"The worst is over," I said. "We find out today if you're through with the chemo."

"We'll be late," I pressed.

"Let's go," I urged.

You sighed and began to sit up. Then you fell back against the pillows.

I sat watching you. "Let's go," I said.

Your eyelids fluttered.

"Look," I said, "if you're feeling so bad, maybe Dr. Choy can do something to make you feel better."

I put my hand over your forehead. It was cool and damp. Your sparse, slivery hair was fine as lanugo.

"Just wash your face," I whispered. "I have your clothes ready for you."

I helped you out of bed. You came out of the bathroom with water dripping down your cheek. I threaded your arms into your shirt, lifted each leg for your khakis. Your loafers looked like blocks of varnished wood on your feet.

I took slow surface streets to the clinic so that the blur and flash of the freeway would not nauseate you further. You grasped a throw-up gambling casino change bucket in your hands. Two withered elm leaves caught on the windshield wipers.

I pulled under the clinic porte-cochere. For the first time, you waited for the valet to open your door, but you declined a wheelchair.

As soon as we entered the waiting room, you fell into the first seat you saw, leaving me to sign you in. You leaned your head back against the wall. The woman behind the desk, your special friend there, looked up at me, then quickly over at you.

"Dore's not feeling well this morning?"

"No," I said. "Awful."

"I'll have him put in an examining room right away so he can lie down."

"Dore?" Dr. Choy whispered on entering. "I had hoped you'd feel like celebrating the successful end of your treatments." She watched you for a reaction but got none. She flipped through your chart, scanned the blood work. "You're dehydrated," she said. "The red blood cells are down again. Let's hydrate you today and give you a transfusion."

It was the first time you would need a wheelchair. The orderly placed your feet on the footrests and began to push you into the hall. The orderly was a tight, compact

Hispanic man with purple lips and fingernails. "Seen this before," he said to you, shaking his head. "They gonna fix you right up, though."

As he was wheeling you from the clinic to the hospital, Kali came up to us.

"I was hoping I'd see you to congratulate you and say goodbye, Dore. It's graduation day!"

"He's not feeling well, Kali," I said.

She was silent for a moment. "Chemo makes a lot of people ill like this," she said gently. "Don't see this as a setback. Now that you're finished, you'll feel better very soon."

The orderly backed you into a cubicle and helped you onto a gurney. A tiny man edged into the cubicle, his head bald as a pecan. He looked like a middle-stage fetus.

"A little stick," he said, as he rolled back your sleeve. I thought at first he was referring to your thin arm, but he was preparing you before pricking you with the needle. You winced. "Vein rolled," he said.

He jabbed again. He hooked you up to the saline solution first. The device whirred; the liquid dripped, filled its cylinder. The device stopped.

"We try other arm," the homunculus said. Then he jabbed you yet again. The device whirred; the liquid dripped into its cylinder; the device stopped.

"Machine broke," the little man said. He went to withdraw the I.V. port.

"Do you have to withdraw that from his vein?" I asked, viewing the charcoal bruises already seeping at both insertion sites. "Can't you just exchange the machine without hurting him again?"

Your eyes were closed. I could see the contours of your skull, your skin dull with a purple-brown underlay.

The little man's eyes started to an unbelievable diameter, as if he were being throttled. He backed out of the cubicle through a slit he had opened in the privacy curtain. An Indian woman entered cautiously soon after. She wore a white lab coat over a yellow sari. She had rouged a scarlet bindi dot on her brow.

"Trouble wid de machine?" She checked the port the man had inserted in your arm, disappeared, reappeared dragging a new machine behind her, hooked you up to it and watched the drops collect in the cylinder, then disperse. A half hour later, she unhooked the empty saline bag, collapsed now like a jellyfish stranded on a beach, added a blood bag. She paused over you a moment and then covered you with a light blanket.

The little man entered to retrieve the broken I. V. machine. He glanced at you, then at me, and winked a prodigious eye. He placed his forefinger to his lips and inched the machine noiselessly out of the cubicle.

I watched you from a chair in the room, glancing at you every time I turned a page of the newspaper. Jeff's obituary was in it: memorial service in three days. No mention of Hugh. I watched your color creep back. I watched your face plump up, the thin skin around your eyes fill in, the veins at your temples recede.

You opened your eyes. They were light-filled, almost merry. "You're here!" you said.

"Where else in the world would I be?"

"I feel better," you said.

"Did you sleep?" I asked.

"I don't think so. I heard you scold that little man."

"Scold?" I asked.

"Maybe not scold, but your tone was certainly stern."

"He was hurting you."

"I'm glad you're on my side," you said.

"I love you," I said. "I was worried about you."

You closed your eyes and stretched, but, remembering the tubing connected to your arm, lay still again. I think you did sleep then, breathing steadily. Your skull receded into living flesh, your arm rounded as I watched: springtime in fall . . . your vernal return.

"Welcome back," I said.

"Ummm," you murmured, your eyes still closed. I fell back into the chair then, restored by this sweet season, however brief, by the kindness all around that caught us that fall.

LAKE TAHOE

We drove to Tahoe one Friday morning to celebrate the successful end of the chemotherapy. An autumnal tartan quilted the foothills. Plum clouds massed over Echo Summit, as if velvet cloaks had remained in the sky after being tossed up there.

We checked into our room at Harvey's. You scored complimentary tickets for a lake cruise on Harvey's restored yacht for the next morning. I swam easy laps for an hour in the fourth-floor pool, gliding as if the water were air.

You stirred from your nap when I keyed the door. I poured martinis. The lake flattened into a sheet of beaten copper; the mountains relaxed. You came up behind me, wrapped your arms around me, and looked out from the dock of my shoulder.

"I am so happy," I said.

"To love!" you laughed, releasing me.

That I could say "I love you" to another person—so freely, so frequently—astounded me. Every time.

I cleared the table in the window alcove. I spread a towel over the table top and backed you onto it. You gazed up at me, then closed your eyes. The mountains crouched beneath a purple sky pricked with stars. We flickered on the glass against the dark world without.

What do I miss most about you? I miss you in your body, its shocking amperage.

That night I dreamed I was falling from the porch of a temple jutting out over a misty recession of distant mountains. I woke with a start to see you dead-still in your sleep. When I caught you breathing, my heart hurtled in alarm at the danger of valuing so desperately what I knew would not endure.

I realized then that love comes with a terrifying risk.

Once in Ecuador, I was hiking the base skirts of Mt. Pichincha with a tourist group, including a woman who had flown from Texas to be with a new boyfriend from her engineering office who had been transferred to Quito. As she reached to take his hand on a down slope, she slipped on some scree and fell, rolling down the path about fifteen feet. I heard the snap of her fibula as if it had been a branch breaking. She was air-lifted out the next morning for surgery requiring a blood transfusion. We stayed in touch. In her Christmas card to me several years later, she indicated that she had contracted HIV from that operation's blood transfusion, one of the first AIDS patients in Corpus Christi. "What a catastrophe love was for me that summer," she noted. Her boyfriend had declined to marry her on learning her HIV status.

At Zephyr Cove the next morning, fifteen invited guests boarded Harvey's restored yacht. You and I stood on the varnished prow, watching the other passengers, most of them elderly, clutch their ways down into the warmer sitting cabin.

Soon we stood alone, balancing on that upper deck in the middle of the choppy lake. The world blenched to blue: water, sky, distant mountains curved in around us like the concave globe of a bubble. I felt I could reach out with my finger nail and burst it. This visible world would fly apart, its arc wince away against the black void it stretched so thin across.

Was it the sudden disorientation of this vision? an unexpected lake swell? a listing of the boat? I stumbled.

"Steady there," you laughed, reaching for me. "You'll fall. You'll break something."

I kept falling.

You caught me by circling my waist in your arm. You leaned us both forward against the cold brass rail that ringed us in in all that blue.

"Steady!" you said. "You'll hurt yourself."

LATE ROSES

"I know you asked for a break after Corey passed, but we could really use you on Wednesday mornings to help with Gary, a client who's just gone on a feeding tube."

I found it difficult to say no. I had no classes on Wednesday mornings. All I had to do was go over to Gary's apartment at about 10:30, disconnect him from the feeding machine which the home-healthcare nurse hooked him up to at about 8:00, flush the tubes, and see how he was. It would take about forty minutes.

"I can do it," I said.

"I don't think you'll be doing it for long."

That Wednesday, I opened Gary's door at 10:15 to hear loud sobbing. I rushed into the bedroom.

"Stop it! Stop it! Stop it!"

Within minutes of the nurse's departure that morning, the feeding machine had clogged and the warning beeper had begun its loud bleat. Gary had had to listen to that beeper all that time, blind from CMV retinitis and too weak to lift himself from bed to shut it off. I slapped the beeper off, flushed the tubes, re-started the machine, held the fleshless bones of Gary's feverish hand while he cried in his darkened room until I could disconnect him. That was my only visit. After I reported what had happened, the Foundation organized professional hospice care.

That evening you were to come over for a light supper after work, then out to a movie. I set out the martini shaker and the stemmed glasses, glancing at the clock.

The doorbell rang. Twice.

You stood in porch light in that early darkness. You had on your dress shirt from work. You gave me a shy, closed smile, shadows pooled dark beneath your cheekbones. You held out your thin hand. These, you said, were the last roses from your yard: a deep-red furl; an orange bud like an amber bead; other small roses, Lenten purple.

"For the bedside," you said. I buried my face in them, gleanings from a fading garden.

"Do you mind if we don't go out tonight?" you asked. "Long day."

"Oh, Dore!" I cried. "Come up and let me feed you!"

GIVING THANKS

"Thank you for being there for me through the chemo. I know the last several months have been rough."

"I'd say the rough months were yours."

"All the same," you said, "I'm grateful to you."

We were sitting on a brocaded banquette sipping martinis. You had asked me to meet you after work. You had reserved my favorite table, the one with a view of the domed Capitol down the palm-flanked boulevard.

"My turn," I said after we were seated. "Thank you for teaching me about loving someone, how to go about it, that it was worth it, that I could even do it."

"You know, we almost didn't happen. I thought you would bail after you learned I had HIV."

"I would have missed out."

The waiter appeared.

"We need more time," I told him.

"Take all the time you need," he said.

"How about forever?" I asked.

"Oh, I'll be back before then."

"I have something else to thank you for," I said.

"What more?" you asked.

"Thank you for making us the greatest lovers of all time."

"What are you talking about? We're greater lovers than Romeo and Juliet?"

"Disastrous puppy-love."

"Greater than Antony and Cleopatra?"

"Political posturers with bloated libidos."

You reflected on this a moment.

I added: "Tristan and Isolde? Their love was spiked by a potion. Eloise and Abelard? She missed out on the necessary equipment for the kind of lovemaking I fancy."

You looked skeptical still. "How about Edward VIII and Wallis Simpson?"

"A Nazi weakling and a divorced American convenience in a Dior gown and a Harry Winston wristlet. Besides, he was a big fruit with a leather fetish, fantasizing about blonde SS troops."

"Sounds a bit like you," you laughed.

"Except for the leather fetish. Now who else?"

"David and Jonathan."

"Okay, maybe them."

"Achilles and Patroclus?"

"Okay, maybe them. Maybe also Rumi and Shams."

"Do we have to compete?"

"We don't: ours is the greatest love story in history, even if no one ever knows about it."

"And love overcomes adversity, which brings me back to what this dinner is for."

"Now about our anniversary," I said, "which is coming up."

"We'll celebrate it in New Orleans at Commander's Palace when I go to Louisiana with you for the holidays. I'm treating, as I am tonight," you said. "Don't argue: it won't be Dutch."

"We'll start off French, but at least one part of that evening will be Greek, I suspect."

"No can do," said the waiter who had reappeared unnoticed. "This is an Italian restaurant."

HALLOWEEN

You wanted to go to the Halloween party benefiting the Sacramento AIDS Foundation.

"It'll be fun," you said, "and I have a killer costume."

I went to Target and the Marts—K and Wal. I did not want to be this year's superhero, cartoon character, ghoul, or—most frightening of all—politician. I went to the thrift stores and pawed through the racks of old clothes. I caught a bad case of the blues, reflecting on the dead people who had shucked these clothes, then on the people whose low incomes forced them to buy them.

I browsed through the costume shops which spring up like mushrooms for a month or so before Halloween in old storefronts vacant the rest of the year. All the costumes smelled like the decayed elastic in an old lady's girdle.

I am not inventive. I cannot sew. And I will not wear a trench coat and flash everyone, as my friend Chuck does every year, showing without shame his sagging old tits.

"Got your costume yet?" you asked me a week before Halloween.

"No," I groaned. "I hate this."

"Poop!" you said.

"Got yours?" I asked.

"Of course," you said. "Told you I had."

"What is it?"

"Not telling."

"Out with it!"

You hesitated. "I'm going in drag! I've always wanted to."

"Is this to be glam drag? Or hag drag?"

"I am going to be be-u-ti-ful," you said. "You'll see."

"Do you have all the stuff?" I asked.

"Melanie gave it to me: wig, skirt, blouse, petticoats, the works."

"Shoes?" I asked. "No way you can fit into Melanie's pumps."

"Oh," you said.

"How about make-up?" I asked.

"Oh," you said.

"Boobs?"

"Oh," you said.

"Oh, Lord," I said.

k. d. lang's new CD, entitled *Drag*, had just been released. lang smoked a cigarette on the CD cover. She had cropped her hair and slicked it back. She wore a charcoal pin-striped suit coat over a white shirt. She looked like an early-stage female-to-male transsexual. The CD title could thus refer to a variety of visual cover references: dragging on a cigarette, cross-dressing. Do I have to explain?

I got it into my head to go as k.d. lang in this recent incarnation. I thought to do a real gender-fuck: I would be a male doing female-to-male drag. Get it? As it turned out, no one else did either.

I borrowed a copy of *Drag* and recorded the title song on a tape player that would fit into the breast pocket of a suit coat. I also borrowed a microphone from my neighbor two doors down, a lonely man addicted to Karaoke. He belted out tunes on his home Karaoke machine each night. You could hear doors and windows slamming shut up and down the block when he started in on "Tie a Yellow Ribbon 'Round the Old Oak Tree."

"Don't drop it," he said. "Don't lose it or break it."

"I'll guard this Karaoke microphone with my life."

"Be sure you do," he said and closed the door on me.

I had the suit already: it had wide lapels and alternating white and black pin stripes on a charcoal ground, all very 1970s. It looked like the bastard offspring of a back-alley hook-up of a zoot suit with a shyster's three-piece.

My hair was a problem. I tried slicking it back like k.d.'s, but I had to slather on so much Dippity-Do that my head dripped. Even then I could feel single hairs slowly loosening themselves from the goo and standing up one by one like intimidated union men exhorted to strike by Gary Cooper in a 30s social-message movie. It was unnerving: it felt as if some arthropod were wallowing around in a tar pit, striking poses for the fossil it would become. So I decided just to gel the hell out of it and instruct it to stand up and take it like a man.

I got to your house and let myself in. You came down the hall to meet me.

"Whoa!" I gasped.

You wore half of an old panty-hose over the short hair that had sprung back after the chemo. You had cut off the leg and tied it off with a top knot. Your lips! Anyone would have thought you had been gnawing raw liver, like Mia Farrow in *Rosemary's Baby*. There were gouts of black liner on your lashes and clots of blue iridescence on your lids.

"Subtle make-up," I said. "Vintage Merle Norman."

"Who are you supposed to be?" you asked.

I pushed the play button of the tape player in my suit pocket. I held the microphone up, leaned back, closed my eyes, and lip-synched the song for a moment, then looked at you.

"Oh, I get it," you said. "Rosemary Clooney."

"Of course not!" I sputtered. "She's old and fat and blonde. And dead."

"Ella Fitzgerald."

"I flashed the photocopy of the CD jacket.

"Ohhh," you said.

"Well, I don't have my make-up on yet."

"That should help," you agreed.

"Your turn," I said. "Who are <u>you</u> supposed to be?"

"A lovely girl," you said. "A signorita."

My eyes widened.

"When I put the wig on, you'll see how it all comes together," you said. "Now let's go attack the make-up for you. I've bought tubes and tubes of it."

"Any left?"

You took me by the hand and led me down the hall. The doorbell rang.

"Better let me get that," I said.

"Why?" you asked, grabbing a candy bowl.

You opened the door wide.

"Trick or . . . ." began a gang of adolescent boys dressed kind of like hobos or like Kurt Cobain. They looked to be about fourteen, far too young to be tricks or gay treats.

Wide-eyed and wary, they eased back from the door. You put a candy bar in each of the bags they seemed too stunned to hold open.

"Freak!" I heard one of them say as you closed the door.

"Don't be offended by that," you said to me. "Remember they saw you without your make-up on."

The doorbell rang again. You swung the door wide open. Your neighbors were escorting their three children on their rounds of the block. The littlest one, dressed like a frog, scooted behind his father's legs. The two older children—Casper and the Little Mermaid—backed off the stoop.

"Uh, is it you, Dore?" their Daddy asked. The children held out plastic pumpkins at arm's length, their backs pressed hard against their parents' legs. His father reached behind him to hoist the frog up in his arms. He turned his green face away from you and buried it in his father's chest.

"Happy Halloween!" you called and closed the door. "This is a blast!" you said.

I put the make-up on. I looked like a more anemic version of you.

You adjusted your wig, a long black acrylic drape. It frizzed out at your shoulders in a froth of curls. You bounced them in your hands.

"How do I look?" you asked.

"Like a goddess."

"See? Told you," you said. "Let's go."

On the way to my car, you stopped to cut a large red camellia, which you bobby-pinned into your wig. It swung out immediately, like a swollen ear.

"I'm Carmen," you announced, adjusting the square yoke of your embroidered Mexican blouse and swishing your red skirt over the black net petticoats. "I'm Frieda Kahlo." You clacked down the sidewalk in loose black flats, the discards of a drag queen who must once have played for the NFL.

You were manic on the freeway. You rolled the window down and yelled at every other costumed car-full driving by. The wig and make-up seemed to embolden you. You yoo-hooed and blew kisses at truck drivers.

"Well, this is a Dore I've never seen before," I said. "Where's my smart, manly, handsome, sexy lover?"

"It's Dora to you, sailor."

You staggered through the lobby in those ill-fitting flats, the red camellia swinging out, then in, like a foliated stop sign. We went up in the elevator to a ballroom transformed into what was supposed to look like a harvest hoe-down barn. Bales of hay outlined a dance floor. Corn shocks and pumpkins were scattered about. A trestle table on wooden saw horses supported several blackened wash tubs filled with witch's brew punch, dry-ice boiling over the rims. An upright black and white cow, rubber udders hanging at his waist, was ladling some into a paper cup.

My friend Chuck greeted us, wearing his trench coat. He started to untie his belt.

"Please do not flash me," I said.

"Is that you, Lu?" he asked, flashing me. "Who are you supposed to be?"

I pressed the play button on the tape recorder, leaned back, brought the microphone up.

"Tony Bennett?" Chuck asked.

"Oh, come on!" I snapped, pressing the stop button.

You tottered towards us with a cup of punch for me.

"Ooooo," gasped Chuck. "What's this?"

"For heaven's sake, Chuck. It's Dore!"

You lunged across me to stick your hand into the fold of Chuck's trench coat, tugging it open.

"Please, not again!" I said.

Chuck obliged you with a quick flash, then stuffed all the sags and hairy folds back into the coat.

Pete, Chuck's partner, lurched up to us. He was a zombie, I guess. He had black eyeliner smeared around his eyes and a bloody gash over his left eye, the same make-up you and I had on, just differently distributed.

"Who are you supposed to be?" he asked me.

I flicked on the tape recorder, brought the microphone up, did my act.

"Connie Francis?" Pete asked.

"No silly. He's Tony Bennett," Chuck said.

"Oh, come on!" I shouted.

You had wandered off. I saw you flicking your wig and chatting with a bearded nun and three hairy-chested cheerleaders in tiny pleated skirts.

Your friend Tim walked up to us. He was dressed as a lumberjack in a plaid flannel shirt, suspenders, and boots. He carried a tiny rubber ax. Otherwise, he looked like he always did.

"Who are you supposed to be?" he asked me.

"Hillary Clinton," I said.

"Don't look much like your pictures," he said. "I don't get it."

"No one else does either," I shrugged.

"But what's with the microphone?" he asked.

"It is not a microphone," I said. "It's a vibrator. Bill is not the only party animal in the White House."

"I thought you were Tony Bennett," protested Chuck, reaching to untie the belt of his trench coat.

"Do not do it," I said. "I mean it."

"Seen it," said Tim.

You clacked over to us, put your arm around my waist.

"Yikes!" said Tim. "Who's this?"

"Tim!" I shouted. "Who do you <u>think</u> it is?"

"No one recognizes me," you whined.

"Foolish mortal!" I said. "You do not know when the gods have favored you."

"I have to tell you in the strictest confidence, Dore, that you are one ugly girl," Tim said.

"In confidence!? In case you haven't noticed, Ms. Lesbian Lumberjack, there happen to be three other people standing right here listening. Lu thinks I'm beautiful, don't you, Lu?"

"I do," I said. "You are Signorita Dora, and I am Placido Domingo."

"I'm confused," said Tim.

Chuck fingered the slit of his trench coat uncertainly, then edged away. He soon returned with a young man in tow, cute enough to eat. He wore a yellow hard hat with a red emergency light twirling on the top, a bulging tool belt slung over tight jeans, a criss-cross leather halter over his bare chest. A sign hung from the halter: Drag Queen Triage.

"Help her," Chuck pleaded, pointing at you.

"Ay-yi-yi," said the young man, assessing you all over. "Smudged mascara? I can fix that. A replacement press-on nail if one lands in the punch? Come to me. I've got wig glue, hairspray, every conceivable shade of lipstick, even half a nerf football I could rig up as a substitute falsie should a boob wander." He stopped rummaging around in the pockets of his tool belt and looked up at you again. "But this," he sighed, taking a step back, "requires more than just a nip and a tuck. I was told a drag queen was in some trouble, but here I find an extra from *Juliet of the Spirits*."

"k. d., this man, or what passes as one, is insulting me," you huffed, turning to me. "Fight with him."

"Will a bitch slap do?" I asked.

"Look, Cinderella-after-midnight," shrugged the drag-queen repairman, "I ain't your fairy godmother. My wand has limited powers. It can't make this come off." With that he turned on his heel.

So the evening went. Someone spiked the punch. Again. The dancing grew frenzied. Your make-up ran. You looked like Marilyn Manson. People came up to you to ask if that was who you were. "Yes," you said, "I suppose I am."

"And who are you supposed to be?" they would ask me.

"Harry Truman," I would say. Or I would say, "Eleanor Roosevelt." Sometimes I would say, "Henry Kissinger" or "Truman Capote" or "John Wayne Bobbitt." Sometimes "Ed Sullivan."

"I don't get it," they would say. "What's with the microphone?"

"I'm Madonna," I would answer. "I forgot."

"That was fun," you said on the drive home. You laid your head back on the headrest. "Did you have a good time?"

I looked over at you and nodded. In the passing street lights, you looked like a terrible ghost. So many others at the party, those masked and rouged revelers who had disguised, for a brief time, the real horrors they faced beneath their costumes, were nonetheless still sick and dying. Like you. This was but a one-night reprieve from the purple lesions still disfiguring under the make-up, the ulcerating herpes sores in the rectum, the parasites and bacteria and fungi and protozoa that had migrated into mortal, now defenseless human bodies from birds and sheep and cats and deer, the various cancers, the haggard emaciations plumped up by the hoop skirts and nun habits.

"Thank you for humoring me," you said when I pulled into your driveway. "Do you want to kiss me like this?"

I held you longer than you expected.

I could not spend the night. I had to be at school early the next morning. I watched you totter down the walk. You pulled the wig off when you got to your door. In the porch light, you looked as you had during the worst of the chemo regimen. The camellia fell in petals onto the stoop. You turned and waved to me and shut the door.

The following year, I went, without costume, to San Francisco with Pete and Chuck, in trench coat, to the Halloween street party in the Castro. You had died the previous June. We could barely make our way down the street through a crush of ghosts, drag queens, Marilyns, bare-chested, black-winged angels. In all that crowd of costumers, I was so lonely for you that I hardly knew who I was.

CALAVERA

When I arrived at Stella's in Civic Center from the BART station, Mary T. and Robert had already ordered cocktails.

"Let me show you what I just bought," cried Mary T., her voice thick with cigarettes and satisfaction. She took from a shopping bag an object swathed in red tissue paper, unwrapped it to reveal a full calavera, a skeletal papier-mache' signorita wearing a yellow plumed hat and whorish red dress, a fold of which she held up by the hem in a ringed hand of bone. Her blank mouth rounded in a hollow lament.

"Marked way down in a Mexican import shop, left over from Dia de los Muertos. Isn't she rich? Don't you love her?"

"She is and I do," I said. I wanted Mary to sheathe the skeleton in its red tissue shroud again before you arrived.

But you did not arrive at all.

"I suppose we'll have to give him up," Robert said, consulting his watch.

"We'd better order," I said a little over an hour before curtain at the San Francisco Opera. "He must be stuck in traffic. I made sure he has his ticket." But I kept turning to check the door, kept noting my watch.

At the War Memorial, still no sign of you. I scanned the lobby for your angular profile in that crowd of dark suits and fur wraps.

We took our seats in the balcony. Your empty chair drew into its vacuum all my fears. The house lights began to dim, the orchestral din rising. And there you were at last, excusing yourself as you squeezed in front of the couple seated between us and the aisle.

"Sorry I'm late," you said and shrugged off your overcoat.

"Everything alright?" I whispered.

You nodded.

"Traffic?"

"No," you said. "I've been in the City for a while."

"Why didn't you join us for supper? I missed you!"

"I couldn't eat," you said. "I didn't have any appetite."

"Do you feel alright now?"

You turned to face me. Your mouth fell open, round and blank, as if you were hesitant to speak. "No," you said. "I took a nap in the car for an hour or so. I feel a little better." The descending darkness of the house pooled yellow in the hollows of your temples and dimmed the red of your tie.

During the long first act, you rested your head on my shoulder. I watched the Valkyries descend and then levitate, big whooping girls on carousel ponies.

During the second act you excused yourself, mumbling apologies as you crawled over the couple at the end of our row. "Stay here," you whispered. "I'm alright." I found out later that you had lain down on one of the benches in the upper balcony lobby behind us.

I see you there, stretched out on that red banquette. You lie face upward in a dim yellow glow, wondering what is happening to you. Is this just an off day, a bad spell? Will you get better this time too? You stare up at the gold-leaf raying through the dimness at the ceiling. Your space is suffused with dissonant music. You cradle your head in one hand, loosen your tie. You close your eyes. Your fever is a fire-ring rising slowly around you, your open mouth a dark hollow in the greater darkness.

"Let's take the elevator down," I suggested after the performance had at last concluded. When you agreed, I knew somehow that you would never again be well.

The stout, arthritic old ladies sharing the mahogany car with us ruffled their furs and shed their heavy scents. You smiled conspiratorially at me and raised your eyes toward the ceiling of the car. We stood back while the ladies ducked their heads to eye the gap between car and ground floor over their bifocal lines, their decrepit escorts bent over gouty and shuffling behind them.

I drove us out of the City, through the trash-strewn streets of the Mission, glass shards gleaming in the car beams. I drove us across the Bay Bridge, your head resting on the back of your seat, the yellow bridge lamps and red brake lights flashing your profile in a syncopation of dark and light.

REGRET

First, Laird.

My initial match at the AIDS Foundation after my volunteer training in 1988, Laird was maybe ten years older than me, short, ferret-like: dark, flat hair that hugged his skull, sallow smudges around squinty eyes. He reminded me of the creepy mechanic in Southern Gothic movies, flicking a switchblade behind his back, blocking the way to the backroom of a filling station with a freezer full of hacked-up blondes. His drawl was swamp-land Georgia, undiluted by decades of post-Navy residence in California.

We always met at my apartment on Thursday evenings. I would cook dinner for us and then we would talk. Or rather, Laird would talk, a white noise of complaints about his clinically depressed partner who sat silent in his lounge chair without moving for hours at a time. Laird felt trapped: he could not afford to move out and go it alone, probably did not have the energy to anyway. And, besides, he did not know how long he had left. He had barely survived a bout of drug-resistant tuberculosis several months before I met him.

After Laird went home, I would pour boiling water over my mismatched thrift store plates and forks, still spooked by the AIDS virus and the TB in spite of all assurances during the training and from Laird that neither the virus nor the TB bacterium could infect me in such casual encounters.

These evenings were, in retrospect, exactly what I had not signed up for at the Foundation. I had signed up for "practical support." This was "emotional support." Naively,

I thought I might offer some suggestions about Laird's predicament that might move him along into some solution. Laird would pause, nod, then immediately return to his complaint, a cud he could not stop chewing.

I realize now that I was there to listen. Just listen.

I went over to Laird's one evening at his invitation to meet his partner, Jerry, a fat, inoffensive man with a breathy voice, a flutter, and a comb over, a pale blip on the radar who would have benefited from a tab or two of speed. I saw also that Laird would never leave. This was it.

Laird and I met for months. Then I bought a house and was overwhelmed within weeks by the scope and expense of the remodel. I saw Laird less and less often: my kitchen was torn out and the house filled with plaster dust bad for his weak lungs. Then even the phone calls trailed off.

Several months later, I got a call from Jerry: Laird had died the night before in the hospital, unable to breathe, infected with aspergillus, a fungal infection of the lungs. In our last phone conversation months before, Laird had said, "I don't know what happened that caused us to talk so seldom, Lu, but it's okay. Make sure Jerry's doing alright when I pass, will you?"

Jerry and I met a week later: dead affect. Flat line. He seemed uncomfortable trying to make conversation. I met with him only that once. I could not figure out what I could do for him.

Laird died and Jerry numbed out of my life thirty years ago. I think I have forgiven myself for abandoning them, though this was perhaps to inflate my importance: mine was a minor role. Nevertheless, my memory of them is stained with a feeling of infraction.

Now Zach.

Regret remains after all these years, like a red wine stain on an often-washed table cloth.

I was one of Zach's many friends. Steven, his match through the Foundation, now himself dead as well, was always there for Zach. I entertained Zach's family at supper on a visit to Sacramento from their farm in Iowa and kept in touch with them with progress reports. I was there to grieve with Zach his decline from pneumonia to CMV retinitis blindness to crippling neuropathy to his final wasting away from disseminated MAC, a mycobacterium that destroyed the lining of the bronchi and lungs. At the end, he was in sporadic dementia. I knew he would not exit from his fourth hospitalization except in a body bag on a gurney.

Steven called me that Saturday in July to tell me that Zach's friends were gathering at the hospital to ease Zach over. I had plans that afternoon to go to a swim party at an old farmhouse just beyond the last Sacramento suburb. The pool, site of porn-film shoots for Falcon Studios, was an exact replica of the outside pool at Hearst Castle, only half the size. In their barn's high hayloft, I would join a group of sweaty men standing around on the hay bales, sex with strangers, late sun aglow in a mote-frenzied haze.

I left the party in late afternoon and rushed to the hospital to find that Zach had died shortly before, his mother on the phone from Iowa begging him not to go. He had been conscious to the end. Zach's left eye remained open despite all attempts to close it.

Regret: the unsettled sensation of inadequate conclusions, a tender spot that aches to the touch of memory: missed chances, selfish choices. Regret, however, differs from remorse, which is all about having done a clear wrong, from contrition for some overt transgression.

My only real regret regarding you resulted from a good intention: I would host a dinner party to cheer you up. I would invite gay men I wanted us to get to know better, like the guys who hosted annual Christmas bashes at a country house so insanely decorated that when they switched on their Christmas lights every evening, house lights flickered throughout the valley and roosters chided each other for having over-slept.

My other guests were a younger couple I had seen casually in the bars for years. They would be one of the first couples to marry in San Francisco when Mayor Gavin Newsome went rogue and granted gay and lesbian couples the human right to marry which we should long have held.

I am a nervous host, fussy to a fault. I spent all day cleaning and cooking and tasting and pothering.

You arrived a half hour early. I could tell on opening the door that you were not feeling well. You wore a gray-striped shirt under a charcoal cardigan. You seemed diminished, your skull prominent, your thin hair slicked back. I noted your dim, pale eye, worry and love and pity and helplessness heavy in me.

"How are you?" I asked, dreading to hear. "You did the Epogen shot today, right?" You had been injecting yourself with this drug to offset the low red blood cell count and anemia three times a week.

"I did the shot, but I'm still feeling puny, but okay enough," you said. "Not very hungry, though."

Everyone arrived at once. Their energy filled the living room, jovial men large in personality. They dispatched shakers of cocktails. You shrank back into one end of the couch. You seemed in retreat; they lowered their voices when they spoke to you.

When I got up to serve dinner, you followed me into the kitchen.

"Let me help," you said.

"Just go sit down, Dore," I said, turning you with one hand on your shoulder and pushing you gently out of the kitchen. "I'll do it."

You walked back into the dining room and took your place. I served the plates, passed the wine, offered a toast to fall, season of passing plenitude.

That night in bed, I held you long, tasting iron.

"I'm sorry for snapping at you," I said.

"You snapped at me?" you asked. "When?"

"When I ordered you back to the table. When I didn't accept your offer to help."

"Oh, that was nothing," you said.

But it _was_ something. What you did not know was that I wanted to be with my guests that evening, not with you. I wanted energy and life and loud male laughter, plates of savory food, strong appetites, wine brimming the glasses. I did not want to worry about you, to be dragged down on this fall evening by pity weighting into my heart so that I began to taste it.

This was the only time I was ever false-hearted or disloyal to you, preferring the company of others to yours, even while you were with me. And though regret is useless at this point, I feel it even now, long after any of this could possibly mean anything to any of us.

HOSPITAL

Through November your appetite made cameo appearances. It came and went. Mostly went. Your diarrhea and fevers grew more severe. Your weight continued to drop alarmingly.

The week before Thanksgiving, a brownish-purple tinged the skin thinning over your skull. You grew listless, uninterested in the life I tried to lure you back to. I insisted you see a gastroenterologist. He looked you over quickly on entering the examining room. "How long has this been going on?" he asked.

That afternoon he put you in a private room on the hospital's AIDS floor, an annex on the oncology wing. "We'll keep you here until we know what's causing the digestive problems."

Once in your room, an IV nurse hooked you up for an immediate hydration and a transfusion. Within two hours, your gold began to glimmer again, darkly grounded at first, like the glinting specks in a gold-panner's wet sand. By early evening, you were already chafing at being in the hospital.

A nurse came in to take your vital signs, preceding the supper cart by five minutes.

"Name's Tiny," she said. I looked the nurse over to gauge her name. She was neither short nor tall, neither thin nor stout. She had breasts heavy to haul around. In a decade or two, they would need to be rounded up and headed out.

"How'd you come by your name, Tiny?" I asked.

"Was a itty, bitty baby when they give me that name. Then I growed up normal-size, but all through high school I got no bosoms, just like little mosquito bites. So just as Tiny was dying out one way, she got started up cruel again."

"I see," I said, giving her breasts a quick once-over.

"These?" she asked, throwing her shoulders back. "After graduate, I come to stay with my cousin Levelle down around Fontana and she know where I can buy me some silicon."

"They're a great success," I said. "What's your real name?"

"Given name's Demoranda."

"A family name?" I asked.

"My momma, she just like it. I put a 'e' to end it."

"To Demoranda?"

"No, to Tiny," she said, levitating her left breast at me so I could see her name pin more clearly: Tinye.

"Tinye, would you please come over to witness what they brought me for supper?" You had uncovered a mess of dark meatloaf smeared in a maroon sauce clotted over a pile of potato lumps.

"Now that do look like the hog's snack," said Tinye.

"Can I order anything else up from the kitchens?" you asked. "I'm supposed to be in here to get digestive problems under control, not aggravate them."

"Tinye, can you oblige him, even if he does think he's checked into a pamper spa?"

"Lemme see what I can do," Tinye said. She returned a half-hour later with a bowl of gluey chicken-noodle soup studded with carrot slices a Technicolor orange, sided by two slices of Wonder Bread.

"Oh for Heaven's sake," you fumed. "I'm going to write a letter of complaint about this to the hospital dietician."

"Meanwhile, Tinye, while Dore is drying out the atmosphere with his outrage, is there somewhere close where I can get him something edible for his supper?"

"Denney's? Over to J Street?"

I brought you back a chicken-salad sandwich, which you did not have much interest in either.

"Request a meeting with the dietician tomorrow," I suggested.

I climbed into bed with you and we watched television.

Tinye knocked before entering the room. "It's on to 11:00. Visitors got to go."

"I am not a visitor, Tinye," I insisted. "I am Mr. Tanner's personal assistant. He cannot do without me."

Tinye's eyes widened. "He famous?"

"Infamous. He's got a bad temper and dangerous connections high up. Do not cross him."

You snorted, undoing all the good work I was doing you.

"Yeah?" Tinye said. "Look close: I be Dionne Warwick taking crap from bad-ass patients like this and their personal assistants just till the dough from my psychic TV channel come rolling in. Which," she consulted her watch, "should be about five minutes after visitors and personal assistants got to leave right now."

You were a terrible patient. You charmed the entire hospital staff and refused to do anything they told you to do. I would arrive to visit you after work, and from down the hall I would hear laughter and hooting and carrying on coming from your room.

Sometimes you visited with other patients on the floor, inviting them in as they shambled down the halls pushing their IV poles before them. Some looked like extras from *Night of the Living Dead*, especially Michael from next door. His partner, also Michael, was bedridden in the same room with him. He died of a raging infection, probably staph, three days after you left the hospital, and his partner, the then still-ambulatory Michael, followed him a week later. Pills and vodka and a plastic bag over his head.

"Get me out of here!" you hissed after these visitors would leave. "Everybody's dying."

You sent your friend Tim and me on nightly restaurant crawls to smuggle something you could eat into your room. On these missions, Tim skulked down the hospital corridors as if he were sneaking into a prison with a saw-blade baked into a pie. I was accustomed to doing the outlaw thing in the open by now. I no longer hid the Styrofoam take-out boxes in the flaps of my coat.

"What's for dinner tonight, you bad things?" Tinye asked when we passed the nurse's station every evening.

Tim blushed and fidgeted with the bag he was carrying.

"Roast beef for that snarling carnivore you've got locked in that room over there," I said.

"Aw, he don't snarl. He purr," said Tinye. "What you got?"

"Tuna salad on rye for me," I said. Tim beat it down the hall.

"Dore tell me you gay guys never mess with no fish," Tinye noted. "He sent back his fish sticks tonight. Wouldn't so much as taste it."

"Come join us, Ms. Warwick. You bring the wine."

"I be fired for sure. Got some grape juice, though," said Tinye, shaking a covered plastic cup.

"That's all I'm asking for—<u>old</u> grape juice—in a green bottle with a long neck."

Your doctors countenanced this nightly contraband. "Whatever he wants," they said, "as long as it's got calories in it. Is he actually eating, though?"

You were in the hospital over Thanksgiving, carping non-stop about the food, the endless tests, the nurses who, according to you, "feel free to come barging into my room whenever they please at all hours of the day and night."

I sat with you on Thanksgiving Day until about 3:00.

"You remove the cover," you said when an aide brought your Thanksgiving tray in around 1:00. "I don't know if I can take what is about to be revealed."

I whipped the beige plastic warmer off, condensation dripping from it. At first we did not register what we were looking at. Then you fell back against your wadded pillows in disgust and flicked the television on with the remote, flicked it off as soon as you saw football.

"Oh my," I murmured, replacing the warmer.

The entire dinner—two thin slices of pressed turkey overlapping mashed potatoes—or was it dressing?—edged by a curdle of creamed corn, the whole overlaid with what looked like putty—was exactly the beige of the melamine hospital plate.

"This is just not right," you moaned, shaking your head.

"Let's just consider this a poorly prepared and particularly unappetizing hors-d'oeuvre. Now try to nibble on it a bit. Think of the starving children in Bel-Air and Beverly Hills. I'll bring you a real dinner from Mary T. and Robert's."

"Please do not force me to view that again," you cried. "The contents of that plate are more obscene than a straight porn film."

I arrived at Mary T. and Robert's around 3:30 for dinner at 4:00. They clucked in dismay at my description of what your dinner tray had put us through.

"I suspect we can make him a plate that might compare favorably," Robert said.

"Put it in a microwaveable dish," I said. "Dore taught me how to pick the lock on the nurses' break room."

"We're going to release him," your doctor told me the Monday after Thanksgiving. "Dore accused me of having put him in Dachau. Doesn't he realize I'm a Jew?"

"But what's causing the digestive problems? What did you find out in the tests?" I asked.

"The test results all came back inconclusive," the doctor said. "I suspect the virus is causing this wasting syndrome, and there's little we can do about that. Perhaps it's some kind of elusive bacterial infection of the gut, difficult to treat, though there are meds for it, like nitazoxanide. But that drug is really tough on the body. I wouldn't want to put Dore through a therapy that would further weaken him, especially because there is no clear indication that crypto is the problem. Perhaps the chemotherapy has weakened his overall digestive system.

Chemo eradicated the cancer, but it may also have destroyed cells meant to divide, like those in his gastrointestinal tract. It's difficult to pin down any one cause."

"That means there's no effective therapy for this?"

"Don't be alarmed," he said, "but we're taking Dore off most of his meds, just until he recovers sufficiently from his digestive problems and regains some strength. Then we'll be able to begin the regimen again, probably after the holidays."

"Oh no," I whispered and looked down at the floor.

"As I told Dore, there's no need for pessimism. He's doing well enough now. We'll start a series of new medications to see if we can boost his digestive efficiency and rouse that finicky appetite of his. His own doctor will see him every week for a while to monitor his progress and to make sure there's some weight gain. Push the calories into him, even when he doesn't want to eat."

"You were unbelievably bad last week," I scolded you. We were back at last in our own bed the night of your release from the hospital. "And you complained about what an impossible hospital patient Bonnie had been after her surgery. Is this a Tanner thing?"

"Survival tactics," you said, "in hostile territory. I am not checking in there ever again. Suffocate me with a pillow first. If you don't, I swallow pills."

CONNECTIONS

I

Shortly before we left for Louisiana, we went to your office Christmas party at the Queen Anne Victorian of your boss in midtown Sacramento. Evergreen swags studded with apples and oranges looped the wooden railings up to the front porch, providing an occasional filched snack for midtown's roving homeless and for the crows dropping down like guilty thoughts from the palm trees lining the street.

In a nod to our Louisiana trip, our host had prepared a Cajun Christmas feast. I have never eaten Cajun food prepared with success by anyone unacquainted with the slither of water moccasins and the rasp of swamp grass. Cajun food, though peasant fare, is more complex than recipes suggest.

"What the hell?" I said to myself after two martinis, "how bad can the food be?"

Edible, all things considered, though the gumbo was watery and a tad on the greasy side: worse, it had no okra, those ribbed pods coaxed from their tan blossoms by hot, humid days and swelling like succulent green penises slow to arouse. (In okra, however, bigger is never better.) And where was the file' that thickens the whole and brings all together like an accordion and a Southern Comfort punch at a fais-do-do?

The break from the antiretroviral drugs was plumping you up. I persuaded myself that the color you seemed to be regaining from your increased appetite would counter the new freedom the virus had to harass your few remaining T-cells, now as rare as debutants at a ghetto rent party.

After dinner, your boss threw open the pocket doors of a double parlor to reveal the Christmas tree, a ten-foot tall radiance. Applause swept the room.

Later in the evening, you and I stood by the tree, admiring it. We were alone together. Suddenly, all light in the parlor seemed to dim. Chairs and tables flew backward out of the scene. The tree too receded. I saw you—singly you—in black and white. No color. No background. Just an emptiness enveloping you.

I have pondered this occurrence often since then, this concurrent vision of gain, of forfeiture; of you present and of you absent. I saw at that moment you centering my life and you depleting it, leaving me simultaneously replete and bereft. As I came in time to understand, this duality characterized our connection in its later phase: having you filled the world; losing you, as I suspected would happen inevitably, emptied it, a duality made manifest in that moment before the Christmas tree.

As suddenly as it had receded, the world rushed in around you again. The severe vision filled and colored. But I still stood outside of it all. I could not find my way back.

You placed your hand on my shoulder. "Too many martinis," you said. "You're cut off."

Your laughter anchored me.

"Are you going to cry now, you silly thing?" you asked.

II

I peered through the oval window at the peaks of the Sierra over the complimentary cocktails brought us by a flirty gay flight attendant interested in hooking up with us in Dallas, where we were not going except to change planes.

"Look," I said. "The mountain slopes indent like the flanks of steers. And the crags look like spinal notches where the bristles rise on their hide joins."

You looked at me from your newspaper, one eyebrow cocked. You leaned over and gazed out of the window for a moment.

"You must have been an annoying child, one of those precocious brats talking forever in a high, squeaky voice."

"Apparently an annoyance to my teachers," I laughed. "My report cards always showed a C in conduct and had two areas checked: Wastes Time and Annoys Others."

"I got all A's in conduct," you said.

"How'd you get so nasty in bed then, Mr. Goody Goody?"

"You mean 'good in bed, Mr. Nasty,' right?"

You reclined your seat and leaned back, your head on the rest. You were happy and warm and, I denied it at the time, already dying.

The Christmas morning vignette of my parents sitting with you at the breakfast table remains with me. You sat between them. Your jade ring had slipped round on your finger so that the band looked like those gleaming on my parents' left hands.

I had been drawn out of my drowsing in the bedroom down the hall by your murmurings. What were you saying to them? They to you? I never knew. When I appeared in the doorway, you and they fell silent and turned to me.

In that pause, my parents' ease with you suggested that the wound opened on their learning that I was gay might have healed at last. Was their approval of you an approbation I still needed from them? Did this acceptance of you as my lover signal a new acceptance of me as well in a way impossible for them before? Until then they could not imagine me as both gay and happy. In some deep place they never shared with me, they still thought of my life as impaired and unrealized. Did they recognize at last that my life could be rich, that I could love and be loved?

When Phyllis and I were living together in Kansas, she came home with me one Christmas. My mother had prepared the guest bedroom for her. I took my old bedroom at the back of the house. "What you do in Kansas is your business," she had told me, "but in this house, you do not sleep with anyone you're not married to."

"Put Dore's things in your room," my mother whispered to me when we arrived. "I've made up the bed for you both."

"I'm puzzled, Mom," I said. "When I brought Phyllis home . . . ."

"You and Phyllis could have married," she said. "You and Dore can't."

III

The day after Christmas, we rode the Greyhound to New Orleans, not needing a car in the city. The bus station gathered the usual knot of working poor, people down on their luck, students with backpacks, and wanted felons. A little black girl sporting twenty different-colored barrettes lay on the station floor crying, yanking at the golden acrylic hair of a Barbie whose buoyant smile remained resilient even in this nightmare kidnapping from the radiant suburbs.

The bus, its toilet ripe, lumbered through narrow streets on the way to the interstate. You gazed out at tumble-down shot-gun houses with sagging couches on collapsing porches and tin roofs orange with rust.

"Even Watts is nowhere near this poor," you marveled. "Compared to this, San Francisco's Mission is Park Avenue."

"In California they tuck migrant worker hovels as bad as this away in fields so on one sees them," I said.

"I'm headin' for Califonia." The words from behind us were a damp purr. I swiveled around in the aisle seat to see a gigantic black man sitting behind us. An incongruity: plucked eyebrows arched over daubs of gold eye shadow, hair napped into short springy dreadlocks gathered on top in a pink elastic band. He laid his hand on his chest, the nails long and tapered.

"Goin' ride this gray dog into the sunset one day," he said. "Soon as ever I can."

"Where in California?" I asked.

"Don't matter, long's I get the hell outta Mamou. Know where that is?"

I nodded yes.

"Nowheres, that's where."

"I imagine it's hard for you living in Mamou," I said.

"Now who goin' mess wit' me? I'm home-growed. I can smite them coon-asses wit' just one black pinkie. Sides, some of them peckerwoods like a little bit of big ole me

167

ev'ry now and agin." He puckered his lips together and looked up at the roof of the bus for a moment. "But I gots to get to Los Angeles or San Francisco, any one of them two. For my career."

"They're far apart," I said, "in different parts of a very big state."

"Where it cool," he said.

"I'd try San Francisco, then," I said.

"Where ya'll goin'?"

"Just to New Orleans."

"Ya'll come see my show."

"What kind of show?" I asked.

"Boy, now look at me. What you think? I gotta say it?"

"Where's the show? When?"

"New Year Eve at Club BangCock."

"Where's that?" I asked.

"It be where you two better come and go in a cab. Les' just say it ain't in no Garden Districk."

"We're only staying in New Orleans a couple of days. We have to be back in Baton Rouge for New Year's."

He shrugged, smoothing a meaty hand up the back of his neck. "Ya'll gon' miss it. Me, I don't do no lip-synch shit. Hell no. Got me a big, high voice like to break glass. I been practicin' till my momma tell me shut up, she like it that much. And I got me a new gown—all shiny gole. Leonard Mae run it up for me. Come see my show. Ya'll like it."

"I'm sorry, but we can't," I said.

He leaned forward and whispered, "How long your sweetman been sick?"

I stared at him.

"Sorrow comin'," he whispered and sat back, nodding. "You be sad."

168

I conned his blank face.

"Good luck to you," I said. "I hope your show goes well."

"Thas' awright. Don't need me no luck." He patted a huge hatbox on the seat next to him. "Got me a new hair, all full up with jheri curls."

"What did he say?" you asked.

"Invited us to see his show," I said.

You looked over at me, puzzled.

"Drag Queen. Big girl," I whispered.

You glanced behind you. "I'd like to see that one in six-inch heels."

"We're invited! Club BangCock."

"No."

IV

I had made reservations for us at the Monteleone Hotel on Royal Street in the French Quarter. My Sicilian grandparents had honeymooned at the Monteleone in 1915 and my parents in 1946. I told you about my family's long matrimonial resonance there.

"We've already had the honeymoon," you said.

"That was all just crazy monkey-sex. We've been together over a year now. This is our anniversary. We're finally getting a honeymoon."

"Anniversary? Honeymoon? I'm so confused," you said.

The morning air wafted the acrid smell of roasting coffee and chicory. I looked over at you lying next to me in our room. One knows the sacred in loving well. Something you taught me: love does bring into accord the animal and the spirit. Bodies, shifting in pleasure, urge souls forward to meet on a high hill and praise again the morning's glow. But the spoiler is there too, the raven that caws across that sunrise. Every time we made love, some part of me disengaged from that pleasure and pondered my vulnerability: a lacerated gum, an unnoticed cut, the virus skulking into an aperture to work its erasures. Sex between us was always pleasure cored in circumspection: we were never to know an abandoned transport. Our loving was a sublimity tethered to care.

I am not one of those gay men who are apparently so troubled by being HIV-negative that they feel challenged by not sharing in their own bodies the viral burdens of their infected lovers or friends. I was never like Noel who defined himself as a "bug chaser" looking for HIV-positive men he called "gift givers." He met his match at a bare-backing party in Los Angeles, an orgy where condoms are not allowed. From this event, he at last emerged HIV infected. I have never shared in the glamour HIV seems to have exerted on gay men like Noel who so readily, even eagerly, submitted to the virus. And Noel was far from being alone in this.

"Now I don't have to worry about getting AIDS anymore," he told me when he shared his new positive viral status. "It's a relief."

I would have given much had you been free of HIV.

When we emerged from the hotel, the morning had dissolved in sunlight. Pigeons bobbed and cooed and strutted like lords on their scaly pink feet. We sat outside at Café du Monde. On this perfect day, you had expanded. You literally looked larger, as if you had feasted on the yeasty air.

I watched the quiet residents of the French Quarter go almost furtively about their daily lives. I observed the psychics and tarot dealers and palm readers set up on the sidewalk in front of the Pontalba Apartments bordering Jackson Square. I would never darken one of those gyp booths: many reasons: a withering skepticism concerning any transaction with the supposed supernatural; a contempt for these shabby dabblers whose own failures to thrive augured an inability to help anyone else into a richer life.

But they had their adherents. I thought I recognized one of them bent over tarot cards laid out by a black woman in a batik turban and bird-skull earrings.

"Matt!" I exclaimed on walking up to him. He warded me off with a raised hand.

"Not yet," he said. "I have to listen."

"Some of these reversals are troubling," said the tarot reader. "Here's the Hierophant. Are you giving your things away again? Are you being reckless with money?"

"Not much," Matt said. "Just a few things to friends, a night or two in the casinos."

"It's not time to do that yet. The cards'll tell you when. Here's the Hermit. Are you getting out, seeing people?"

"When I feel up to it."

"You need to get out. Look at Temperance reversed: hostility, frustration. You're not that sick."

"Damned doctors," Matt said. "Damned clinic. Damned insurance."

We eased away and returned to our table at Café du Monde. "I went to school with him. LSU. We graduated the same year. English majors."

"Here he comes," you noted.

"Sorry guys," Matt said on approaching us. "My weekly session with Claudine. I didn't know you were still around, Lu. Looks like you finally came out. Who's this?"

After introductions: "I tried teaching English for a while after the M.A. I got from Loyola. Then I got sick. Pneumonia. You know the kind. Liked to killed me. Then swollen lymph nodes. Thrush and Esophagitis. Night sweats that nearly drowned me. Then sores supposedly caused by cat scratches even though I don't have a cat. My T-cells went to hell, stayed there too long, and got roasted to cinders. It's all a bitch. And people tell me I'm lucky to still be here...."

Matt looked over at you: "But then I suspect you might know something about all this."

I bought Matt coffee.

"Tarot, Matt?"

"It makes as much sense as anything else in my life. Besides, Claudine tells it like it is, unlike all the bullshitters I meet at the clinic."

"So how's Jacques?" I asked, cautiously.

"Who? Oh, <u>Jacques</u>! Funny how freaked some people get by the virus. Swore he'd stay with me, then up and left. I got back from Baton Rouge to see my folks one weekend and the apartment was empty. I see him around from time to time, but what's there to say?"

"You know, I always liked Jacques," I murmured.

"Yeah, me too. Look, gotta go: talking about the past gets me down. You know: missed chances, wrong turns and all."

"I hope that didn't upset you, Dore," I said as Matt walked away with a strange rolling gait and leaning on a cane. Neuropathy, I suspected.

"How could it not?"

V

We returned from New Orleans to spend New Year's Eve with my family at my brother Damian's house outside of the antebellum town of St. Francisville. His house sits on ten acres of the Port Hudson Civil War battlefield, an important site in what I was taught as a child to call the War of Northern Aggression.

The last day of 1997 was cold and dark. Rain fell in swaths of gray through the pecan trees.

The bonfire after dinner was a soggy affair. The wet logs, doused with kerosene and lit, sizzled and hissed grudgingly into a respectable blaze at last. It had stopped raining. We fired off rockets and Roman candles. Explosions flared and ricocheted through the woods: I imagined the ghosts of Confederate soldiers rising to arm the trenches, believing they were mustered up again, Yankees in their midst. We were home by 10:30.

"Be careful on the roads, tonight of all nights," my father called out as we left for George's, a gay bar. We would see the New Year in with our kind. We put on plastic tiaras and sipped cheap champagne bubbled up by bar backs dressed in diapers with 1998 sashes across their bare chests. We tried to evade the smeary kisses of tipsy revelers.

"May this be the best year ever in all our lives!" I whispered through the midnight din.

We woke late. We made love quietly. It was so silent in the house that the rustling of the sheets sounded to us like hand claps.

"Is your gay card current, Mister?" I asked, incredulous in the Blockbuster video store after a family lunch when you told me you had never seen Bette Davis in *Hush, Hush, Sweet Charlotte*. "We cannot let another moment pass."

"I liked it well enough," you said as the VCR whirred in rewind, "but I don't see what all the fuss is about."

"Liked it!? Fuss!?" I spluttered. "You hopeless fag! Are your really gay?"

"Let's take a nap," you said, shrugging.

"First you must be lessoned," I said. "I saw that movie in early high school and queered it right away. Bette Davis as Charlotte was a projection of gay little Lucien. She's trapped in that crumbling Greek Revival closet of hers with a haunting secret. She's persecuted by her purring cousin in heterosexual league with someone Charlotte thought to be her advocate."

You stared, obviously not convinced.

"Finally, in a revelatory moment, she finds out she wasn't really who people persecuted her for being, that the role of deviant had been foisted on her by others until she saw herself that way as well. You gotta love that great final scene where she comes out at last from her columned antebellum closet dressed in that to-hell-with-you hat, fitted suit, kiss-my-ass pumps, fumbling with her clutch and gloves. Curious bystanders murmur, 'She don't <u>look</u> crazy!' What a great paradigm for coming out! For a little Southern closeted sissy queer boy with no role models, that movie was *This Is Your Life* in code."

"You were thinking all this when you were fifteen?" you asked.

"Earlier."

"It was a great movie, Lu. I loved it."

"Figured you might."

After our nap, we went out for a drink with Pat and Jerry. With Pat I enjoyed my first relationship in the 1970s, that era when I was so hoping to be straight, even against all counter-signs. With Jerry I spent several cold, muddy, hungry days of marijuana and music at Woodstock in 1969.

When we returned to the house, my mother was nodding in her chair. My father suggested that she get ready for bed. She looked up vaguely and closed her book. Then she struggled out of the deep chair she had been sitting in and started out across the room, her slippers slapping the hardwood floor. Suddenly, in mid-stride, she started to tilt. You and I both leapt up to catch her. She fell against you but hit the floor hard.

"I'm alright," she said, breathless.

We lifted her cautiously to standing position.

"Does anything hurt you?"

"My leg. Not bad," she said.

The next morning we learned that she had sustained a simple fracture. I decided I had better stay on a few days longer in Louisiana.

"Aw," you lamented, "you won't be on the plane to tell me that from the air the oil holding tanks at the refineries look just like white polka-dots on a brown dress?"

"Just drop me at the terminal," you insisted when we arrived at the airport.

Our holiday was over, our connections aligned: co-workers, family, acquaintances, friends.

"I'll be home soon," I said.

"Hurry!" you said.

THE PLUM GROVE

I

I watched you sleeping, huddled on your side, your mouth open on the pillow.

I crept through the house, wrapped in a blanket. In the backyard, a mourning dove clattered to the fence, its flared tail edged in silver. The air deepened to orange, then suddenly whitened. I looked over my shoulder to see you blinking in the kitchen, white light showering down on you from the skylight. You seemed to dissolve in it, as if you were glass. You held a blue Marinol pill in your open palm.

"I cannot take any more of these," you said.

We had sat up together most of the night after you had taken your prescription for this pharmaceutical cannabinoid given to increase your appetite. You had been so stoned and anxious you could not lie down or even sit still.

"But you'll take the other new drug, right?"

"I'll try," you sighed.

AL-721 was a drug given to start the appetite, encouraging weight gain while alleviating diarrhea. It seemed to have little effect in restoring immune function, nor did it help to control the virus. It was a thick, oily, orange substance consisting of fats extracted from egg yolks and mixed with other lipids. It smelled ghastly and tasted worse. I juiced an orange and spooned in some sugar, then mixed the crud to thin it as much as possible. You delayed when I called you. I kept stirring.

"It's the snot-curdle of hell," you said. You stood over the sink, staring out of the window for a moment. Then you took a sip and swallowed. You took another sip, gagged, spit it out.

"Breathe deeply," I coached, my hand on your shoulder. "Relax first. Then down it quickly."

You shrugged my hand off. You took a deep breath. The glass tilted up and up. When the glass was on the counter, you were still gulping.

"Good," I said. Then you vomited it all up into the sink.

You had begun taking the antiretroviral drugs and protease cocktail again, Crixivan this time. These bouts of nausea were flushing the pills out of you before absorbed. Within two weeks, your doctor would take you off these meds for the last time.

"I need to rest," you said.

"I'll be back around three or so," I said. "Anything you want from the grocery?"

"Whatever you think best," you said and closed your eyes.

What to buy? What to tempt you with? I had memorized all the grocery shelves by then and the meat, seafood, and bakery counters. Every time I went to the grocery, I tried something new that you could fix effortlessly for lunch. These items were stacking up in the cupboards and freezer. Your appetite was as shy as a fawn abandoned in an oak dapple.

I got to your house about 2:45. You were sitting up, showered, shaved, dressed. Your hair was slicked back like a 40s matinee idol. You looked pleased with yourself.

"I feel good," you said. "I slept through the morning. What'd you buy?"

You wrinkled your nose at the raviolis. I put the carton in the freezer with the other rejects, a cold company of Siberian exiles. You were gracious to the game hens, distant with the ground meat.

I opened the slider to air the house and then sat with you. Your body seemed a second-home to me: your long torso and the deep divot at your throat, your perfect teeth.

I suggested we take a walk in the late light now gilding the window screens. The neighborhood was spuming in flowering quince and Bradford pears. You surprised me by agreeing. You had not been out of the house for several days.

"We won't go far," I assured you. "Just to the grove of blossoming plum on the corner."

We approached the grove from the east. The sun was a dilated brilliance behind the plum trees. Petals flushed as they fell. You walked into that radiance, the slant beams transfiguring you. I stood on the perimeter of the grove: branches, blossoms, your body all now dissolved in light.

I stumbled into the grove, blinded. A moment or two passed alone in a dazzling silence.

"Dore!" I cried. "Where are you?"

Suddenly your arms extended around me from behind.

"What is it?" you asked. "What's wrong?"

"Don't leave me," I said.

"Of course not, you silly thing." You pivoted me to face you, golden light raying around you. "Did you think I went home?"

I held you in that golden air slow chilling around us.

II

After supper, I martini-dozed in front of the TV but woke to your restless flipping channels with the remote. You were sitting up. The furnace was roaring.

"Is your fever amping up? Are you sick?" I asked

"I don't think it'll be bad tonight," you said.

I got another blanket for you and the kidney-shaped basin we had taken from your hospital stay at Thanksgiving. I put my hand to your forehead.

"Don't fuss," you said.

The siege was brief. You did not vomit. The fever spiked but soon settled down. Then you paled and grew cool to my touch.

"Ready for bed?" I asked.

You shambled down the hall.

"This old body is falling apart."

"I love each piece," I said. "I'll close up."

I went to check the front door. The moonlight beckoned me out of the sweltering house. I stepped onto the stoop and stood surveying the yard. The shy daphne planted by the door respired a cold sweetness up from snail-shaped purple buds.

The houses were all dark down the block. I walked again to the plum grove at the corner. The flower haze had now gelled into white marble, black-veined by branches. Heavy clumps of blossom were hoisted up as if for some suspended construction in the air, marble blocks levitating to converge.

In that white stillness, my heart suddenly failed me, overwhelmed with fear. I put my hand out to steady myself on a plum branch. The tree swayed, the whole frozen white mass of it.

A possum snuffled among beer cans in a recycling bin set out curbside. A shuddering chill compelled me back to your house, across that silver spill and through those black shadows.

Moonlight angled in through a bedroom window, dimming the red plaid of your pajamas. The hand laid on your chest glowed silver from wrist to fingertips. Your mouth had fallen open, a thin, dark crescent.

I lay beside you. You nestled closer. You murmured a few faint notes. I saw years ahead reliving this moment.

"I love you," I whispered.

"Love you, too," you sighed and drew your thin lips over to warm my cheek.

CANCELLATION

"I'll send my donation in, and I'll call John to tell him I can't come."

"Something's come up at work?"

"No."

"Are you ill?"

"Not ill, no."

"Then what? Why are you canceling?"

A long pause.

"I just don't want to be in a crowd tonight. I don't want to hear a political speech while jammed up tight into a corner of John's living room. You go. Then come by later."

I went to the fundraiser alone. I tried to reach a table spread with crackers and cheese cubes on a tray. I found myself jammed into a corner of John's living room listening to a campaign speech by a lesbian running for a seat in the state assembly. Domestic partner legislation. Republican threats to reproductive rights. Funding for breast cancer research and women's health. AIDS. Gay adoption issues and parental rights.

I was edgy without you. Your standing next to me would have made the fundraiser bearable, even without food, without a drink.

Jostling my way through the crowd, shoulder-tapping a passage toward the front door, I made my escape. Ben, a neighbor of mine, was standing on the front steps, smoking a cigarette and sipping wine from a plastic cup.

Ben's recovery from meningitis had been remarkable. Three months ago I had received a call from him: he had been throwing up all afternoon and had a headache so severe that he could hardly look down or move his neck sideways. He was disoriented.

"We're going to the emergency room," I said. I suspected it was meningitis. I had seen this before. I had had to have a meningitis vaccination.

We waited in the ER for over an hour even though I shared my suspected diagnosis with the in-take nurse. During that time, Ben was increasingly incoherent, mumbling and agitated. At one point, he slid from his chair and lay on the floor. A nurse came over to him but apparently determined that he was in only ordinary distress. "I think it's meningitis," I told her again. "I think you need to get him out of the waiting room."

Others in the packed waiting room edged away from us. When at last a nurse called Ben's name, he was unable to respond. Orderlies helped him onto a gurney. They admitted him. They started an immediate IV. They kept Ben for several days, releasing him to his house two doors down from mine. By then his sister had come up from Fresno to stay with him. Now he was drinking wine and smoking. He looked great.

Not for long, as it turned out. Several months after seeing him at this fundraiser, Ben called and asked me to join him in meeting some friends for Sunday brunch served by drag queens at a local gay bar. When I met Ben at his door, he looked like gray hell, holding onto the door jamb and weaving.

"We've got to cancel," I insisted. "Your friends will understand. They can come over here later."

"If you won't take me, I'll drive myself."

When we arrived at the bar, Ben's friends were waiting for us on the sidewalk. Ben fumbled with the car handle, finally managed to open the door, and sagged out of the car face down onto the tar of the parking lot. His friends piled him back into my car and followed us to the hospital emergency room.

Ben never left the hospital. Several days after he died without regaining consciousness, I noticed Ben's brother-in-law loading a large U-Haul with Ben's possessions.

"Ben left a list of bequests," I told the brother-in-law, who did not pause in his loading of a box of dishes with my name written on the side of it in Ben's hand. I had helped Ben compose the list and had promised to see that his things went to those he had designated to receive them.

"Yeah, we found the list. Ben was out of his head. We tore it up," he said as he continued to load other objects on Ben's bequest list into the U-Haul.

"Lucky you," I said to Ben at the fundraiser. "You got a drink."

"Rot-gut Chablis from a twist-top jug," Ben scowled. "You can always tell, no matter what fancy decanter they pour it into."

"I guess the idea is to pull in some money for the candidate."

Ben rolled his eyes: "Another lesbian with a fish-stew agenda. Not my zoo; not my monkeys."

"Still," I said, "those issues concern gay men too. Those who want to control women's bodies want to control our bodies as well."

"Say, what's with Dore? He told me he was coming with you tonight. I saw him walking on the Mall at lunch today. He looked terrible, so pale, so thin."

"Did you tell him that?" I asked in alarm.

"Well, I was in shock."

SCORING

I am agree with this topic. . . . .I scan the essay this sentence introduces and score it a 4.

In morden wold. . . . . This essay earns a 2.

Ferstival, I say with sagacity that. . . . . a 3.

I am scoring an essay test which assesses the English proficiency of international students whose first language is other than English. The test is being scored in Emeryville, a town at the flat lower join of Berkeley and Oakland, just before the San Francisco Bay Bridge on-ramps.

I have been attending these occasional weekend readings for many years. The honoraria, though modest, and the camaraderie of colleagues from across the country combine to make these weekends pleasant diversions from the routine of the teaching term. On reading weekends, I would leave for the hotel on Thursday evenings and return to you late Sunday.

On Saturday evening immediately after that day's reading, I bolted down three glasses of merlot at the scorer cocktail party and was asleep by 6:15 with the alarm set for 9:15. I awoke in the dark to the static of an untuned radio. I arrived at the Steamworks soon after, roamed the seedy backstreets of the Berkeley flats for a parking space, and walked in a cold drizzle to the line forming at the base of the stairs leading up to the reception window.

I do not like standing in this line on the street with these men sizing me up, me eyeing them back, transgressive in our gathering in outside, heterosexual air. Here, we breach the strict breeder code we usually take such self-protective care to observe in public. Inside the baths, however, we display our desires openly in gay space, without shame or danger. In that humid arena, channeled gay need erupts in free sexual expression at last, liberated from its cramping in the outside world.

I turn to the wall when cars pass, though it would be wiser to face the cars in case they carry gay bashers armed with paint-guns or burned-out neon light tubes or bottles filled with gasoline or battery acid, the bastards. Once inside the stairwell and off the street, I relax, though I am impatient with the gossip and slow processing of the towel boys behind the window admitting the regulars in line.

"An hour and a half wait for a room," I am told at the window.

"Just a locker," I say.

I hand a twenty through the slot in the window. The towel boy is pretty, a clear 9, so I do not protest when he slips my two dollars change into his tip jar without my offering it. He gives me a card to fill out, much like a hotel registration. I indicate my name as Dorian Hallward, the first of my attempts at anonymity in this place where one sheds one's personal identity, where one simultaneously objectifies and is objectified.

"Been reading Oscar Wilde, Dorian?" the pretty towel boy asks. He informs me he is an English major at Cal.

I step into a dim foyer. The white towel I am issued is still warm and smells of Clorox. Soft-drink machines splotch the foyer in red and blue auras. Several men in towels sit on a bench scoring the new arrivals, stage-whispering and laughing. As I walk by them, I overhear a consensus number for me: it is a 7. It is my evaluation score out of a scale of 1 to 10. A "C," I think": adequate, average, acceptable looks. It is the score I would give myself. I would give the loud, nelly one in the middle of the bench a 5—five for fat and giggly—the other two both earn flat 6's. The guy standing by the water cooler, however, scores a clear 8. But he is not looking at me. He is gazing through an open arch into the television room at a lean, youthful blonde watching a porn film, his Pepsi perched on a frayed sofa arm. The blonde knows he is being cruised. He is in no hurry to engage. He is a 9.

The upper half of the foyer wall is open so one can look down into the locker well and watch the new arrivals undress. Bathhouses offer the erotic consolations of voyeurism. They untether gay gaze and nominate it witness of naked acts. All is uncovered. There is no hiding here; the closet is turned inside out. Here is the anarchic refusal of gay desire to relinquish or retire.

Two men are changing in the locker room when I enter: a young Asian who looks far too boyish to be there undresses under the interested eye of an older man who is buttoning his shirt. He is gray and balding; his black plastic glasses are too large for his face. He has apparently stopped off for a quickie after work as a realtor holding a Saturday afternoon open house or maybe after Saturday vigil Mass, but at 10:15, it apparently took him longer to get off than he had hoped. He is on his way home to Kensington or San Pablo with excuses to a wife who probably no longer much cares to hear them. He is a 4.

The young Asian man is attractive in a way I am not attracted to, too young, too short in stature, someone else's 8 maybe. He eyes me sidelong as I take off my shirt. He stalls, messing around in his locker to appear busy. I take off my jockey briefs. He glances at me, his eyes migrating up and down me.

"It cold tonight," he says, his English so burdened by his first tongue that I do not understand him right away. Then I wonder if he is making some kind of allusion to the fact that I am flaccid, balls shy.

"It cold!" he says again. He is Chinese, maybe Vietnamese or Cambodian.

"Yes," I shrug, "but it's warm in here. Soon it will be <u>hot</u>!"

He gets it. He laughs too hard. "<u>Hot</u>!" he rasps, trying to growl sultry. "Yeah, <u>hot</u>!"

He introduces himself: "Raymond."

"Really?" I ask. "My name's Lu."

"'Lu' mean 'beautiful' in Chinese," he says. What does 'Raymond' mean in Chinese?"

Raymond looks baffled for a moment, then laughs. "Horny," he says.

I climb the stairs out of the locker room, my white towel cinched around my waist. I am enveloped in a techno-music throb: no words, just gasps and moans syncopated with a relentless beat as if from some mechanical heart. The long hall pouts in dim red light, like infrared.

Raymond makes no secret of trailing me. Every visit I make to the baths, I seem to attract young Asian men. "That's because Asians revere the elderly," my friend Chuck offers when I notify him of this. Raymond is persistent: he wafts his hand lightly over my chest as I edge by him, leaning against a wall. I am not a rice queen, the sobriquet given gay Caucasian men who lust after young Asians.

I walk the halls. I recognize men with obvious HIV: protease inhibitors often produce telltale deformities—the lipodystrophy of "buffalo humps," or fatty deposits that swell the nape of the neck up into the mastoids; "ropey legs," or depletions of fat in the lower extremities, resulting in protruding veins spiraling up over gaunt calves and thighs; overly distended abdomens in otherwise lean, muscular men.

A man in his early forties stands at the end of a row of rooms. Something in him arrests me: he is not as handsome as you, but a hint of you strikes in him. He is darker than you; though not hairy, hairier than you. Perhaps his hair, darker and wavier than yours, is highlighted like yours used to be. I gaze at him, a sexy 9. He glances at me, glances away.

Raymond has come up from behind and positions himself across the narrow hall and just down from me.

"It <u>hot</u>!" He attempts a sexy snarl that sounds like throat-clearing. He laughs too hard.

I look at the attractive man down the hall. He looks at Raymond. Raymond looks at me. We are deployed in a triangular misalignment of lust. I edge past the handsome suggestion of you and hook his eye. No response.

I plod down the endless hallways studded with doors. Is it even desire anymore that keeps me, bored, winding through these red corridors? I tell myself that I am here because I love the radical democracy of bathhouses: one cannot tell Ph.D.s from janitors, high school dropouts from Silicon Valley CEOs. The clientele blends all shades and races, all castes and cliques, though tonight there seems to be a disproportionate number of Asian, African-American, and Latino men, perhaps because these cultures are largely unaccepting of homosexuality, the baths thus providing a place of safety for these men to indulge their tastes. Also, these men may not have the financial resources to maintain private apartments or houses where they can entertain other men. Fine by me: I am an equal opportunity homosexual.

In the bathhouses I experience a strange, revolutionary freedom accompanied by a withered joy, perhaps because I suspect that I am here to search for sexual approval, for the lift of being desired without any real pressure to satisfy that desire. And I find myself willing to take that pleasure in the admiring overtures offered me by anyone—the old man with a belly so ripe it has bifurcated at the navel like a peach cleft (a 3); from the guy with muscular dystrophy, who negotiates the halls with a steel crutch, mouth distended by the effort (a 5); from the effeminate black man with the high, shelf-like ass swishing from side to side as he walks (a 7)—it doesn't matter. I reap others' yearning, garner attention, harvest approval— the fodder that feeds me desirable. This may be the real reason I find myself here, why I endure this withering tedium.

But this is not the only reason. My time is getting long here. A man lying on his back in his dim room moves his head to follow me whenever I pass his open door. He is purple in the red light, in his forties, at least a 7, maybe an 8. His black hair glints silvery and sexy in the shadows. I pass the open door again. Again he follows me with dusky eyes, lifting his head from the cupped hand it rests on. I linger against the wall opposite his door. We size each other up. He is slender but soft in the gut. He has an appendectomy scar slashed maroon along his lower belly. He motions me in. I close the door behind me and mumble my first name. I do not get his clear—I think he says "Carlos."

I like the way he frowns at me as I fuck him, a hard glinting eye to eye, his head raised, his mouth a fierce rectangle, breath harsh and rasping. Suddenly his eyes roll to the ceiling. His mouth goes dark and taut. He comes with a groan. After a moment, he puts his hands out against my thighs and pushes me away. I slide the condom off and drop it on the floor.

He raises himself on one elbow. "Did you come?"

"No," I say.

"Do you want to?"

"That's okay," I say.

I stand.

"Let's hook up again sometime? Do you live in the East Bay?"

"No," I say. "I'm in the area on business." I open the door. I step back into the room, lean to kiss him quickly on the lips. "That was great," I say. "Really great, Carlos."

"It's Luis."

In the showers, I stand under the hot jets and soap myself. Another man in the showers watches me, masturbating.

I go to sit in the steam room, busy with group grope and blow jobs. The old guy sitting next to me reaches over and begins to play with me. I let him. Then he leans over to put me in his mouth. I put my hands on his hairy shoulders and gently push him away. I stand to leave. "Bitch!" I think I hear.

I lower myself into the steaming chemical soup of the hot tub, a square pool tiled in dark blue. Raymond is there. I do not look at him. I base my head on the pool rim, inhale the fumes from the vat I am steeping in. The strong chlorine scent is the smell of the city-park-pool dressing rooms of my childhood, boy eyes roaming with impunity over the bodies of fathers undressing, their largeness of hands and bodies and penises my initiation into desire. I wrap my sodden towel around me. I head to the place I knew on entering that I would end up.

I climb onto the catwalk ringing the glory-hole pit where the cocksuckers stalk. Several men stand around on the catwalk with me. A man in his fifties, a 5 or 6 I would say, stands next to me. He has trimmed the brindled hair on his barrel chest short and bristly. He runs his hand over my abdomen. I let him. He licks the flat of his thumb and rolls it over my left nipple. He nuzzles my neck. A hand feathers my right calf, gently tugs me over to the railing. I look over to see the man with the leg brace smiling up at me, leaning on his metal crutch.

He lifts my towel and takes me into his mouth tenderly and holds me there. Then he slides me all the way in, gently extrudes me. He moves me back and forth, rhythmically. I throw my head back, close my eyes, lean into him. The sliding accelerates. The barrel-chested man steps behind me, flicks my towel off and drapes it over the railing. He bites my ear, fingers my nipples. He tries to fuck me, but I push him away.

I shudder, gasp. I try to pull out of his mouth, but he reaches a hand up to grab my ass and jams me in as deep as I can go. I can feel him gulping. He slides his mouth up and down on me, then slips my cock out and kisses it. I open my eyes, look down over the railing. He is smiling up at me. He kisses my cock again and cradles it in his hand, so gently.

I shrug off the barrel-chested man who is still playing with my nipples. I squat down and kiss the man in the leg brace, a quick kiss. He cups his hand behind my neck, closes his eyes, opens his mouth. I pull away.

"You're the best," I say.

"I liked it too," he says. "A sweet payoff for a job well done!" He smiles crookedly. "Come see me again," he adds. "I'm like the bank—always open for deposits."

In the showers I soap and soap myself. I let the water gush over me for a long time. The soap smells antiseptic, like oleander sap.

I walk the corridors naked back to the locker room, the towel too wet to bother wrapping it around me. I open my locker, place my shoes on the bench. I turn my underwear right side out. A young man with short dreadlocks is undressing before a locker three down from me. He sports a tiger tattoo on his left arm, shadow on shade. He is a 7. My watch says 1:36 A.M. We eye each other.

"You done?" he asks.

"Yeah," I say. "It's a wrap for me."

"Another time, then."

"Maybe," I say.

"Anybody around?" he asks.

"You'll have an easy time," I say.

"Man, I don't want me no 'easy time.' I want me a good, hard, dirty fuck."

"It'll happen," I say.

"But not wit' you. Look: I don't want me no fag boyfriend. Just let me do you right here and I can go home."

"Next time," I say.

"Yeah, shit," he snorts and brushes past me, cinching his towel.

The air outside is thick, foggy and cold. The glistening streets are deserted. I sprint to my car, looking over my shoulder. Bad neighborhood. I drive the black freeway to the lighted hotel. Catholic-grounded as I am, I think of the moral implications of where I have just been, of what I have just done. Is it right to use someone who wants to be used, who obviously takes pleasure in being used, who offers himself so willingly, so eagerly, who, in turn, is using me in exactly the way I wanted to be used? Isn't there a reciprocity there, a kind of mutuality, in a way a kind of instant and satisfying intimacy, even affection, however temporary?

In my room, I take another shower. I fall asleep instantly.

Sunday's reading goes smoothly. We finish by 3:00. I arrive at your house around 5:00. It is already dark, though a cold copper outlines the western horizon. I stumble over the morning papers still on the stoop and fumble my key in the lock. The house is silent and dark. As I close the door behind me, I hear a rustling in the family room. You are lying on the couch, shrouded in a blanket, the basin teetering on the edge of the coffee table, within easy reach. You raise yourself halfway when I enter the room but then ease yourself down again.

I switch on a lamp.

"I missed you," you say.

I am shaken by your appearance: a large-eyed meagerness narrows your face. Your skull seems to be pushing through, taut, sallow skin protesting. On my return, I find you brittle and sunken.

You had had a nausea attack with high fever and chills late Saturday afternoon. We had grown practiced in dealing with these, but this was a particularly virulent one. It had frightened you, alone in the house. Your fever had spiked to 103; you could not stop vomiting; the chills wracked you so that at times you had to fight to breathe.

You had called a friend of ours and asked him to stand by in case you needed to go to the emergency room. He had done exactly what you had not wanted him to do: he had rushed over, had stayed and hovered when all you wanted was to be quiet and still, riding out the nausea heaves. He had fussed and worried and made noise and lit lights. You had finally persuaded him to leave, with thanks, late Saturday night after you lied in assuring him that the attack had subsided.

"I'm here now," I said, and caressed your cheek.

"I'm so glad," you said.

I brightened the house, made a light dinner for us. You had not eaten since Saturday morning. I watched the color begin to return as you downed a few mouthfuls, drank some Gatorade. I washed the dishes and scrubbed the pots and cleaned the kitchen while you riffled through the TV Guide, calling out program options to me.

I propped myself up with pillows against the arm of the couch. You lay between my legs, your head resting on my chest, directly over a heart ever true to you, ever faithful.

LIGHT BREAKFAST

Often I would ambush you in the kitchen when you rose in the mornings, welcoming you back to life. Staggering from my exuberance, you would submit under the kitchen skylight. Your hair rayed in glassy tines. I could read your ribs like braille beneath the white blaze of your t-shirt. Ingratitude was never my failing. Those kitchen mornings I would clasp your ebbing, big-boned body in my arms in thanksgiving.

For several weeks, your appetite had left you in the lurch. Nothing would entice it back. Before packing up and leaving for good, it had skulked around surly for months. Occasionally I could tease a tidbit before it that would make it sit up and take notice. But now, nothing. You observed mealtimes out of custom rather than need. You seemed beyond food. Worse, when your appetite decamped, it made off with your energy as well. We never saw either ever again.

Every morning I asked what you wanted for breakfast, out of habit, out of hope. Oh, you did not know. Well, no, no more oatmeal. Or cereal. No more eggs, toast, bacon. No more waffles or muffins or pancakes or biscuits. No more fruit smoothies or protein shakes. For sure, no more Ensure. Farewell to earth's abundance.

Sometimes I would juice an orange, stir in a small amount of protein powder you did not see me add, and hand you a glass full. You would sit up on the couch and look at it. "It glows like a jewel," you would say, holding it to the light. You would sip it, then set it down. "You better drink it," you would say after an hour or so. "It'll go bad."

"You have to <u>eat</u> something!" I would sometimes cry in a blind fugue of frustration and despair. "Are you not eating on <u>purpose</u>?"

You would meet this anxious scolding with downcast eyes and a slight sigh.

Many mornings you would say maybe you wanted a pink grapefruit, to quiet my plying. I would overlap the grapefruit slices in a fan pattern to please your eye. After sifting sugar through a gleam of sunlight, I would lap the juice up over the pleats, glazing their pink bittersweetness.

This morning grapefruit routine repeated day after day after day? How wearying morning after morning tending to you in a silent frustration, worrying over your inability to eat. "This is how I spend my time," I would sometimes sigh: "I peel bitter fruit for a man who cannot eat it!" Though carping, I consumed myself in a fervor to serve you, anxious to see you take food and chew it, flushed in pride and pity when you finished at least a quarter of the bowl!

On one of these mornings, you came over from the couch to sit at the counter. My wrinkled fingers were stinging in the acrid juice dripping from the grapefruit segments I was arranging. The curves of your lips, thin and gray, upturned tired. I placed the bowl before you. You smiled, the grapefruit shimmery in the skylight's white glow.

"Let me say a blessing," I offered.

You bowed your head over the bowl, your wan face flushed in an up-splurge of pink light.

"May this fruit fortify you. May its sweetness and light illuminate the dark where the virus coils. May my love that sets this fruit before you strengthen you to stay with me always."

"Amen," you said.

"Let me feed you!" I blurted, taking up a spoon.

"Not yet," you said. "Not yet."

You took the spoon from me. You dipped and lifted it, freighted and radiant.

WHEELCHAIR

I

We stood in the doorway, peering into the dark corner where Peggy said it was. She fumbled around the door frame for the switch to swing the garage door open, rarely raised now that Peggy had given up driving. The door convulsed up, protesting like an old man in a rest home roused for a visit by a worthless grandson looking for another cash handout.

The chair sat collapsed like a shriveled spider. Snared in rips of dusty plastic as if trapped in its own ruined web, it lay waiting for you, folded up long ago after the death of Peggy's cerebral-palsied son Jamey.

I backed the chair out of the corner. It rolled easily, though wreaths of plastic wound among its wheel spokes. The foam of the handle grips had dried hard and brittle, scabbing under my palms. You sat next to Peggy on the driveway in the white-wicker chairs I had lugged out for you both from the backyard. I stood between you, the three of us eyeing the wheelchair now standing in the sunlight, Lazarus called forth and blinking back at us.

"The goddamned thing's a mess," Peggy rasped. "I should've gotten it ready for you, but I'm old. Go to the side of the garage, what's-your-name, and you'll find a bucket and some rags next to the spigot."

I tried to open the chair by tugging the handles away from each other.

"This one's no goddamned mechanic," Peggy coughed. "Pull the arms apart, you, and it'll open."

"Looks a hell of a lot better," Peggy said after I had sponged the chair down. "It cost a frigging fortune when it was new. My Jamey had to have it: he called it his Rolls Royce." She cackled. "That Jamey was a hell of a crackup. Remember that boy of mine, Dory?"

"Of course," you said. "We grew up together."

"He's gone a long time now," Peggy sighed.

Had I required a wheelchair, I would have met the mischance with bleak resignation at best, more likely with resistance. But you were as unflappable as I would have been upon acquiring a second-hand bicycle to ride to work on. Indeed, when I first suggested you might want to use a chair—"just for those times when you want to save your energy"—you agreed so matter-of-factly that I was astonished.

The wheelchair glimmered with chrome spokes and wheel rims. Blue tubular steel framed the undercarriage. A red-and-white sign hooked to the rear bumper of the undercarriage proclaimed "God is my Co-pilot," at the bottom of which Jamey had scrawled, "but I'm doing the driving, so watch out! Even God's scared!"

You detached this and handed it to Peggy. "You might want this," you said.

"That Jamey: always the goddamned jokes!" Peggy croaked. "I used to laugh till I peed my pants. He'd run his hand over his face a few times and go all bashful when I told him he ought to gone on Johnny Carson."

"Hop in!" I said. "I'll take you for a spin."

You lowered yourself into the sling seat cautiously. I wrestled with the foot-rest attachments.

"You got the goddamned things ass-backwards," Peggy roared. "Reverse 'em. See? Yeah, like that. And put the brake on while he's getting in and out of the chair lest he fall and bust his skinny butt."

"Got to tell this one everything," Peggy confided to you, as if I had already left.

You sat still while Peggy and I fumbled and fussed. I released the brake, pushed the chair back and forth a few times. Then I wheeled you down the driveway to the sidewalk, gaining speed.

"Wheee!" you said dryly. "Here I go!"

Lifting the chair into the car trunk proved a cumbersome task: it was bulky and barely fit into my Honda Civic. It would slide in only one way.

Driving back to your house, I looked over at you. You stared straight ahead.

"I've come to this," you said in a voice without expression.

Your laugh surprised me: it sounded as if coerced by some lame, inappropriate joke.

II

"I'm falling out of my clothes," you complained one day as I was stripping the bed to wash the sheets. You had just showered. You were sitting in your jockey shorts on a bedside chair in a wedge of sunlight. "I don't have anything to wear anymore. And those sheets are frayed and stained."

"Let's go to Macy's tonight, then. Downtown?"

You took a deep satisfaction in using the handicapped placard. You directed me into a parking space adjacent to the elevators, a "Doris Day parking space," like those she pulled her white convertible into, always right at the door of her destination in those perky 50s movies she made with closeted Rock Hudson.

"Do you want to use the chair?" I asked.

"I'd better."

This surprised me: Macy's downtown crowded so gay that it was as cruisey as the bars. One shopped the Men's Department for a date for Saturday night.

You stopped the chair at a rack of khakis and pulled two pairs off their hangers. You propelled the chair with your foot over to short-sleeved shirts, riffled the rack, chose two, both blue. You picked out a brown belt. You directed me over to the cash register.

"Don't you want to try them on?" I asked. "Did you adjust sizes from what you used to wear?"

"I'll try them on at home," you said. "Of course I downsized. Why do you think I'm here? Shoes next."

You seemed oblivious to the gay men all around us, fingering the clothes and eyeing the prospects. You ignored their quick takes, inferences announced on their faces. Some tried the normative gaze, as if you were invisible. Others looked away quickly. Some prolonged the gaze, seeing in you the specter of AIDS gliding among them, some of them infected too, others relieved not to be. You wheeled heedless through, ignoring the men negotiating around us. Past all that.

I wheeled you to linens, your lap filled with shopping bags. You wanted 400-count Egyptian cotton sheets and pillowcases. You liked an Italian Renaissance-patterned counterpane in lavender on a white ground. We added a white cotton blanket.

"Did you enjoy shopping?" I asked you on the drive home.

"Not really," you said after a long pause.

"I love the things you bought," I said.

"Shrouds. Winding sheets." You looked away and laughed.

"Why wait, given the circumstances?" you said that evening when I asked you if we should use the new sheets to make up the bed. You sat blinking in the lamplight in the chair beside the red cabinet. You put the Macy receipts in the black-lacquered bottom drawer of the red cabinet.

Three wide bands crossed the counterpane. Renaissance urns laden with fruit, vegetables, and flowers charged the middle band: pears and clustered grapes, tendrilled gourds, roses and sunflowers. In the lower band, Greco-Roman dolphins finned past other fish on stylized waves, each supporting a putto, his cheeks swelling at the spiracle of a conch shell. In the upper band planets danced, each conducted by its guiding spirit. Saturn twirled at the touch of a maiden, her long fingers plinking its rings. Mercury whirled on the thumb-and-forefinger fulcrum of a sylph.

I stopped spreading the counterpane and let it settle. I sat on the edge of the bed, my back to you.

"I know this wasn't your first choice," you said after a moment. "But do you like it?"

"I do," I said, not yet able to look at you.

"Everything's there," you said.

"Everything," I said, "and you centering it all for me."

Several months later you died on the sheets you chose. I had you buried in a pair of khakis and one of the blue shirts you purchased that evening. I had the white cotton blanket laid loosely over you, even though it was early July.

III

Water from last night's storms sparkled in the redwoods and folded each new liquid amber leaf around a glittering bead.

I let you drowse for a while. Soon you came out to the family room.

"It sounds like a riot out there!" you said.

We peered at the patio to see magpies tossing worms which had wriggled out of their sodden burrows. On the lawn, the mockingbirds and the scrub jays had renewed their turf wars, screaming and counting coup. And a gathering of pragmatic sparrows pursued their ruffling and twittering, discussing the day's construction projects under the eaves.

"It's life out there," I said. "Let's go out into it!"

"Where do you want to go?" you asked. "I don't want to go far."

"How about we take the chair and I wheel you down the bike trail along the American River between the Watt and Howe Avenue bridges? It's a little over a mile."

Shortly before noon, we drove to the river. Several gay men—or married men from the suburbs with certain tendencies—were already cruising the parking lot, leaning against their cars or sitting in them reading the paper.

I lifted the wheelchair out of the trunk and carried it to the asphalt bike trail. We started slowly.

Clouds skylarked in the upper air, which was as fresh as all of spring itself. I glided you past golden California poppies and the just-bluing spires of lupines. Squirrels scolded in the cottonwoods among quivering leaves of the palest green glass.

You looked directly before you, neither to the left nor right. I stopped once to ask how you were. I stepped to the front of the chair. You closed your eyes against the sun and lifted your face to me. The flesh had failed on your cheeks, pooling at your mouth in a rubbery roll. The light dusted your sketchy hair.

We entered a dark defile on the path, a cut through a black-walnut grove. Mossy boles sprawled above us, blown slant or undermined by a fractious river prone to disregard its banks. We entered this damp glen down a gummy mat of last fall's leaves. Then we both smelled it at the same time: something—deer, coyote, raccoon, jackrabbit— something had crawled into this glen to die.

"I'll get us out of this!" I said. I pushed the chair at a fast clip until I was running. We whizzed along.

"Go back, not through it!" you called. But I was already careening up the incline, a lucid opening just ahead. We emerged in sunlight, the sick-sweet fetor still in our nostrils. But the spring world quickly renewed itself around us. A flock of orange tanagers foraged in a thorn hedge just leafing out to the river side of the path.

I wheeled you to a stop at the trail end of Howe Avenue. We looked out over the access parking lot, at a Mexican family, the flap of their red pickup down to brace food tins being laid out by a tiny abuela in black, mariachi music blaring.

"We should head back now," you said.

"I'll get us through the bad stretch quickly," I said. "Hold your breath when we enter."

I paused above the defile, rallying before entering the dead zone.

"Maybe we should just stop delaying it, Lu, and get it over with."

I ran us through the valley, the death stench clinging to us. Once through it, I continued to run. You moved your hands from your lap to grip the armrests. I ran through a whisper of new leaves, the world wheeling by us. To fill my lungs with this new air, scented fresh now with honey locust, to move exuberantly again! You looked back up at me once, then turned forward. I ran and ran, rolling you through the spring. I stopped only when we reached the car, my pulse bucking.

"How was that!" I panted.

You did not answer. You took your hands from the armrests and crumpled them together in your lap.

"Ready to go?" I asked.

"I'm a little dizzy. Let me just sit for a while."

"Too much? Too fast?" I asked.

You declined to go out again in the chair for a ride along the river when I invited you on future days even finer than this one had been.

IV

Through March you worked mostly at home. I would hear the computer whir on, then the rapid click of your fingers over the keys sounding like a Doberman prancing across a parquet floor. You were writing a report about some state division chief fingered embezzling from the agency she headed. Occasionally you had to go into the office. You declined to use the chair on office days.

One morning in April, you came into the family room where I was reading the papers over coffee.

"It's decision time," you said. "I just finished the project I've been working on for the last month. The office has approved the report. I'm done."

"So what's the decision you have to make?"

"Whether or not to give up my job."

"But you love your job," I said. "What does the Bureau think?"

"They want me to stay, even with my erratic hours in the office. They'll work around them."

"And you?"

"I don't know. I hate to keep calling in sick. I need to think it out."

"Let's go to Tahoe," I said. "A road trip will allow you to talk it through with me on the way up."

We climbed into the mountains. The wheelchair rattled in the trunk. Mounds of blackened snow crusted the sides of the highway.

"They realize I can't come into the office regularly," you said. "And I can't go into the field at all anymore. But I'm one of the most experienced report writers they have. They want me to stay on and work at home."

A silence settled over us.

"And I really want to stay on," you said. "At least for a while longer."

"That sounds to me like a decision."

At that, we rounded the point where Highway 50 descends into Tahoe, the azure lake below us. Boulders jutted over the roadbed, their lichen a Chinese-lantern orange. The lake spangled through the bay window of the high room you had booked at Harvey's.

"How do you feel?" I asked on returning to the room after your nap and my laps in the fourth-floor pool.

"Good!" you said.

"Good enough for a martini?" I asked.

"A third of one."

I threw back the curtains. We watched the mountains belly up to the lake as if to drink there. The water flinted steel, then relented in a soft maroon.

"I'd better use the chair tonight," you said as we left the room.

After dinner, you wanted to gamble. I wheeled you slowly up and down the line of blackjack tables. Finally you chose. The dealer's badge named him Dylan. He was obviously gay but with a hard edge: he looked as if he had recovered from some recent illness, AIDS-caused, I suspected. His hard red hair fell over a defiant brow capping collapsed cheeks. Life had conned him once, and he would be damned if he ever let that happen again. He had drawn the wrong hand and had played it badly, but he would amend all that. His mouth pinched in creases as if he wanted to spit out a sour phlegm. But he dealt the cards with poet hands.

You started to win from the first deal. Dylan's hands glided like sylphs. You won and won. I held the new handle grips of your chair, peering over your sparse hair at your winning hands, beginning to doze standing up.

"I want to play a bit longer," you said. "I can get someone to wheel me back to the room if you're ready to turn in."

From a sound sleep, I heard you slide your key card in the lock. I sat up to see you push the wheelchair before you.

"Why didn't you get someone to wheel you up?"

"I leaned on the chair handles. It's no big deal," you said.

I lay down again. You sat on the edge of the bed, running your fingers lightly through my hair. I drifted asleep. I felt you cup my body into the curve of yours. You slipped your hand under my pajama bottom.

I turned to you. "Did you win?"

"Oh, yes."

"Let's sleep," I said. "Breakfast is on you."

You rolled on your back and laced your fingers over your chest. I raised myself on one elbow. "Tomorrow?" I asked. "Is that okay?"

You had wended a slow way through dim corridors, leaning on your chair to reach me sleeping in our room. I am sorry now that I was not open to you then. Love comes to us so rarely, even hobbled. It strikes me now as unwise ever to turn it away.

And why did I not take you into my arms? A waning of desire: the diarrhea, the wasting, the fevers and chills, the aching bones and joints, the bouts of nausea countered that longing for you that had so long ruled me.

But I loved you at that moment in this declining as much as I had ever loved you when we so often tore the bed apart and flung the pillows to the floor in that slippery joy when my desire for you could not be stilled, when, within minutes of the quaking, I coaxed you for more. I loved your abated body on this night as much as I had ever loved it when I wore it close as my own flesh. Maybe more. Love, I learned, grows ever more steadfast the closer it comes to death.

"You are not concerned about me, are you? About meeting any sexual needs I might have?" I asked over breakfast.

"I wanted you," you said. "No more than that. It doesn't matter."

"I love you," I said, taking your hand.

The Keno girl saw this and skirted our table.

V

The road to Virginia City rose gradually. The high hills crowding this Nevada silver town marbled the blue hue of aged beef. We were there for a day's excursion from Tahoe.

I rumbled you over the rough boards of the sidewalks in Virginia City, past the souvenir and t-shirt shops squatting in 19th Century frontier facades. You storked wearily through the Mackay Mansion with its funereal Victorian settees and portraits of leading citizens stiff with a rectitude tarnished by the 110 saloons and brothels in this Mother Lode town during its 1870s silver mining boom.

"I think we might want to get back," you said around noon.

"Don't you want some lunch before we leave?"

"I feel a little sick from thumping over the boards in the chair," you said.

"How sick?"

"I'll manage," you said. "But let's go back."

"Pull over!" you cried as we drove down the main street out of town.

"Here?" I asked, eyeing the sidewalk filled with tourists.

"Pull over! Pull over!" Before the car had stopped completely, you had opened the door and vomited into the gutter. People walking the raised sidewalk shied back.

"Let's go," you said.

We drove maybe two miles.

"Pull over!" you gagged. You vomited on the side of the highway into spindly blue wildflowers, cars whizzing past. When you were breathing normally again, your head on the headrest, I suggested we stop for a break, that perhaps the motion of the car was worsening the attack.

"I want to get back to the hotel," you said.

Down the road a ways I could see a casino. I stopped for five plastic coin buckets and a clutch of moist hand cleaners. Every time you vomited into a bucket, I gagged. Between sieges, your head lolled from side to side on the rest, swaying at the whim of the road. I cranked the car heater on to combat the chills.

When at last we reached the hotel, you declined the wheelchair. I watched you shamble heavily into the lobby, clutching a plastic coin bucket. I had never seen this leaden hefting before. I returned to the room to find you in bed with your clothes on under the counterpanes of both beds, the heater roaring through the grates.

"Just leave me as I am," you protested as I unbuttoned your shirt and slid your pants off, coins spilling out of your pockets.

I sat on the edge of your bed in that darkened, sweltering room, listening to you pant, your teeth chattering. You were awake, your eyes closed, concentrated, as if in a test of wills with the nausea. At last your eyelids fluttered open. You looked at me a long time without saying anything. What is there to say when the worst is happening?

"You're better now?"

You nodded, almost imperceptibly. You peeled the top counterpane away, and I removed it to the other bed. You turned your face to the wall and slept. I sat with you for a long time. When I rose from the bed, you opened your eyes.

"Feeling better?" I asked.

You nodded.

"I'll let you sleep some more. Do you need anything?"

Your head nuanced no on the pillow.

"Then I'll go do a few laps in the pool."

You nodded and closed your eyes.

After my laps, I sat in the hot opal whirl of the spa.

As soon as I entered the room, I could tell something was very wrong. The dark silence tensed with it. Then I smelled it, an antiseptic reek, Lysol leagued with a cloying rug cleaner and a room deodorizer.

I sat on the edge of the bed. I laid my hand on your cheek and drew it away, scalded by your hot sweat. But it was not sweat. It was tears. You suddenly clenched in sobs, shattering, guttural. I have never heard anyone weep like that, before or since. And I cried too. I sobbed with you in that terrible darkness.

"What happened?" I asked in a pause. "Tell me."

"I couldn't make it to the toilet in time," you choked. "I fell. It splashed on the carpet and up the walls. I was lying in a puddle of it. It was so violent that I couldn't control it. They sent two maids in to clean it up."

I lifted you to sitting and placed your head on my shoulder. I held you, smoothing your back.

"There's nothing to be ashamed of," I whispered.

You started back suddenly. "I am not ashamed," you hissed. "I am not ashamed."

I settled you to me again. You rested there, weeping more quietly now. Never again did you ever abandon yourself like this. When you had quieted for a time, I laid you back on the pillow and turned on a light.

"The two maids spoke only Spanish," you said. "I gave them each $25. Do you think it was enough?"

"I think so, yes," I said.

"They worked fast. They were finished in ten minutes."

"They wore gloves?"

"Yes. They threw my underwear away. I had crawled into the shower before they came to the room."

"Then it's done."

"Does it smell bad in here?"

"It smells like the restrooms at the bus station just after the custodian has mopped through, maybe a bit like a port-a-potty."

"Oh, great."

I sat by the bay window staring at the plum shine on the water. I read for a while, glancing occasionally in your direction as you slept. This marked the beginning of a constant monitoring, a straining to catch your breathing, a watching for even an involuntary twitching at the borders of sleep.

Then the television flickered on. You began to channel-surf with the remote.

"This may strike you as a stupid question given the events of this long day, but are you at all hungry?"

"'Hungry' is a word that's lost meaning for me. More like 'empty'."

I read you the room-service menu, interrupted by your calling out correct Jeopardy answers to Alex Trebec. You clicked past many channels, your food tray ignored in your lap. Finally you handed the remote to me.

I stopped at the History Channel's report on the McCarthy witch hunts. We watched the doomed Roy Cohn shadow the brutal senator, ever at his ear. Cohn would go on to die of AIDS.

"We gay people have our villains," I said, "just like everyone else."

"Some say Cohn deserved his end," you said. No one deserves this, I thought.

"Let's go home tomorrow," you said quietly.

In the morning we drove over the high passes through mists obscuring the peaks and valleys above and below us. We followed the center line of the road down.

"Tomorrow I'll give it up," you said. "I'll go to the office to tell them. Can you take me?"

"I can," I managed.

VI

"Why don't you come?" you asked, flossing your teeth in bed.

"It's your day," I said. "I'll dilute the focus. You'll have to contextualize for me everything you want to talk about. You go. I'll take you and pick you up."

I had ached enough loss: your hair, your health, hearty nights of lovemaking, now your job. I had seen enough cards tossed into the box.

You looked as if you had borrowed an older brother's suit. You slicked your hair straight back in the handsome way you had taken to wearing it. You looked clean, polished, urbane, and very ill.

I rounded the car down the parking lot spiral into your numbered slot underground. I started to lift the wheelchair out of the trunk.

"We're close enough to the elevators," you said, a hand on my elbow.

"Dore," I called after you. "Will you be alright? Do you need me there?"

"No, I'll be fine."

The early-May day blurred with a blue rain burdened with bus exhaust. Homeless people muttered like damp crows perched on planter rims all along the K-Street Mall, their grocery carts cloaked in black plastic leaf bags.

I pawed through Macy's sale rack, fingering fall and winter clothes in their seasonal demotion and sizing up the men descending the escalators.

"Lu!" I heard. "Is that you?"

A face I did not recognize materialized from the other side of the rack.

"It's Hal. We trained together at the AIDS Foundation years ago? I was the receptionist there later?"

"Hal?" I ventured. Had the lithe blonde man I once seriously lusted after shifted into this grim apparition in so few years? "Hal, I almost didn't recognize you!" That graceful head, profile by Phidias, had bloated: mastoids had thickened and neck had humped so that upper back and skull had fused. Strong chords bracketed his collapsed mouth. His abdomen bulged. The protease inhibiters Hal was obviously taking rescued lives but often wrecked looks in a brutal exchange.

"I think I saw you recently at the doctor's. I was leaving as you were wheeling your match from the elevator. He didn't look so good."

"He wasn't my match. He's my partner."

"Oh, sorry!" Hal said. "Who was he?"

"He isn't a client of the AIDS Foundation. Actually, I'm hanging out waiting for him. His retirement luncheon is going on right now. I'm picking him up when it's over."

"He was still working?"

"Let's get together for coffee sometime. It's been far too long, Hal," I said.

"How about now?"

"I'm expecting Dore to call any moment," I said. "You have the same number?"

"Wait a minute. . . . That was Dore? Dore Tanner?"

I wanted away from Hal's past-tense verbs, darting at me like hornets.

The call came for me in housewares.

"Bring the chair up," you said. "I tired myself out."

You were sitting in the office lobby, a white Styrofoam container in your lap, the lunch you could not eat. A paper grocery bag by your feet held the last few items from your desk. Your co-workers stood around you, talked out and awkward. They watched me help you into the chair before embracing you in clumsy hunches over it and wandering off to their cubicles. Your boss stayed behind.

"Thank you for everything," you said to her, your voice unsteady. "For all the years. I'll never forget what a great job I had. I always looked forward to coming to work."

Your boss took your hand, gazed at you a moment eye to eye, then put her cheek to yours. "You did good work, Dore. We'll miss you."

When we got back to the car, I helped you buckle your seat belt. When I got in, you reached over, and with your thumb, you erased the tears tracking down to where taste reminded me how bitter they were.

VII

Bonnie accompanied you to your final Friday doctor appointment. I was scoring papers in the Bay Area. She wheeled you into the examining room. After the ritual we had realized there so often together—the weighing-in tolling yet more weight-loss, a review of medications, the cold stethoscope and the crackling blood-pressure cuff— this time your doctor leveled with you: if nothing were done, you would die within ten days.

You wept. Your gaunt legs dangled from the examining table. You lowered your head between hunched blue shoulders and cried quietly, tears dripping between your knees, two knobby cudgels, your chest heaving, shadowed a sallow purple, plucked goose flesh. After a moment, Bonnie laid her hand on your upper arm to feel the grief shudder through your bones.

So you consented at last to my fervent, insistent pleading, to what you had so long protested you would rather die than accept: a feeding machine. There on the dark margin, at my urging, you determined to claim a little more time. Did you condemn yourself a coward in this approach of the death you protested you did not fear? Did you judge you had flinched in the dark face-off?

This I know: you elected life, however limited, however brief. You tacked away from dissolution, not out of fear, but from an ardent election of existence, each fraction of it. You chose life with the certainty that you could fend death off for only a short while, enough time for a few sunset drives with me along the delta in the LeBaron convertible, the loved world farewell-reeling before your tired gaze, the wheelchair left at home.

Your decision buoyed us both during the following days, though not so wholly but that during the nights, dismay and doubt sometimes seeped into that darkness.

Several mornings before the scheduled surgery to install a gastric tube, you needed a transfusion. I wheeled you over the glass bridge from the hospital to the lab in oncology. In the middle of the bridge, suspended over the street, we met Dr. Choy. You had not seen her since the conclusion of your chemotherapy treatments in the fall.

I braked the wheelchair.

"Dore?" she said. "It's been a long time!"

"Not so long," you said, your voice breaking. "I'm not doing well."

"I'm sorry," Dr. Choy said. She extended her hand to touch your shoulder. She left it there a moment, then slowly withdrew it. "I'll tell Kali I saw you."

I bent over you. "You beat it," I said in your ear, almost a hiss. "It didn't win. You did not fail."

"What would you know about it?" you asked, your tone flat, words raspy as fallen leaves.

SIGNIFICANT OTHERS

I

After that final wheelchair visit to your last transfusion, we were granted several more months for you to live, or, as you might have termed it, several more months for you to endure. You were growing more and more weary, more and more frail. Alarmed by your evasiveness about your health in those final months, your brother Tom and sister-in-law Ginny would not be put off any longer. Your brother Joe drove over from the Bay Area to join Tom and Ginny for the Sacramento visit. Bonnie was here already because I had grown apprehensive about making health and financial decisions for you. You were spending whole days on the couch or in bed. Bonnie joined me in trying to persuade you that portions of the world were still edible.

You protested this family gathering. "It's a death watch, a hover," you complained. "I'm not there yet."

As if on cue, your siblings disguised their dismay at your decline. "He's a shadow of himself," Tom whispered to Bonnie in the hallway.

Soon after their arrival, we called at the Sacramento AIDS Foundation to see about getting home health care assistance for you. "I don't want you to have to bathe me," you had said to me a week earlier.

"But why not?" I protested. "You know I can do it." I had given up working as a volunteer at the Foundation when you got sicker.

"It's because I want you for my lover, not my caregiver."

"But I can be both!" I said. You shook your head and looked over my shoulder at the wall opposite. "You already have too few rewards in our relationship."

The Foundation put you on its list of clients. It was unlikely, the caseworker cautioned, that we would get any immediate help. The client list was lengthy, the staff roster short, funds scant.

On Thursday afternoon, Tom cut the grass, the mower thrumming under the eaves, droning more distant by the sidewalk. When the motor spluttered silent, Ginny told me Tom wanted a word with me. Tom was sweeping the sidewalk, leaving green swaths of grass stain on the concrete.

"We wanted you to know how grateful our family is to you for being such a good friend to Dore," he said.

"A friend, yes, but more," I insisted. How singular it is to talk to straight men about what they often are conditioned to find repugnant. One listens for the false note, watches for a curl of distaste at the lip. Straight men may on occasion have to defend their choices of whom they love, but never that they love. How can an intense gay love ever be expressed to a tall man not pausing from his sweeping?

Tom nodded, stubbed the toe of his work shoe at the dried slime shell of a crushed snail. "Dore's not doing well, is he?"

"Not at all."

"How much time do you think he has?"

"He could still turn it around," I said. "Others have with the new meds that are coming out."

We still had some hope then. Or I did. You progressed through your days as if you had some secret plan. Nothing suggested a defenseless biding of fatal time. You would regroup. Who more deserving than you?

Bonnie listened silently to my repetitions of all this. On one occasion she interrupted, "He's dying, Lu. You need to understand that."

"He'll rally!" I said, more loudly than necessary. "They'll start the antiretroviral drugs again soon. The doctor says so. And new ones are coming out all the time."

Soon after, Rhetta Sproul, your caseworker at the Foundation, arrived at the house. She hugged a brown clipboard to her chest, her breasts splaying out to either side of it. As she walked, her panty hose rasped. A tiny voice warbled up from that abundant source. You eyed her warily. You inched up in recoil as she approached you, her extended hand fleshy as a catcher's mitt.

Apparently Rhetta's assessment was dire because the Foundation acted sooner than we thought, sending over a home-health-care aide within two weeks of her visit and coinciding with the departure of your brothers. The aide would work from 10 A.M. until 2 P.M. several days a week.

The aide was a nursing student from Zaire, Columba Ogeebee, who was supplementing her government stipend working for the AIDS Foundation while studying at U. C. Davis. I have never seen anyone blacker: her skin absorbed light like a black hole. Her hair was hidden in tied swaths of gold and maroon cloth that framed a small, heart-shaped face. Her clothes seemed to float in air, moved by an animated absence. She spoke in a voice accented like the cooing of doves.

Her presence in the house signaled a repugnance at the prospect of even ordinary living. She threaded her long fingers into latex gloves on the stoop even before she rang the doorbell. She scowled askance at the laundry piled by the washing machine. After her first attempt, we relieved her of any obligation to bathe you. I watched you dip yourself into tepid water. Columba doused your hair with a plastic cup. You shivered, your back goose-pimpling. She splotched shampoo in the center of your head and worked it in with the tips of fingers sheathed in latex.

Columba stayed with us three uneasy days. I had determined to call Rhetta to tell her not to send Columba on Thursday when Rhetta herself rang up to tell us that Columba had resigned from the Foundation. Columba could not, Rhetta reported, work with AIDS patients after all: her father and an older brother in Zaire had both succumbed to the disease. On her last day with us, Columba had picked off her latex gloves as she left the house and balled them up in the mailbox.

"We're sending out Julia Droop," lilted Rhetta in her doll-baby voice on the following Monday. "She'll be permanently assigned."

"What's she like, Rhetta?" I asked, cautious after Columba.

"She's just starting with the Foundation. Her interview went okay. One thing: she's not the brightest star in the night sky, but she should be fine."

The next day, I heard a car stop up on the curb in front of the house. From the car radio, Madonna belted out what she thought a virgin might sound like, then abruptly shut up. The yellow Camaro's right front was crumpled like a wad of newspaper, the headlight goggling out of place and held on with duct tape. A woman sat in the driver's seat, staring straight in front of her. After a couple of minutes, you joined me in spying from the kitchen window.

"What's she doing?" you whispered.

I shrugged.

The woman snapped open a black vinyl purse big as a picnic cooler, unfolded a square of paper, looked at it, then at the house. We ducked back from the window. When we looked out again, she sat staring straight ahead, her hands on the steering wheel, absorbed as if seeing a vision of the Virgin Mary materialized on the windshield.

At last we heard a car door slam. I opened the door to her ring.

"Julia Droop?" I asked.

"Been a long time since anybody call me by that name," said the ginger-colored woman blinking up at me with the tobacco eyes of a golden retriever. Rusty freckles spotted a face framed in bronze wisps escaped from a topknot yanked up onto the center of her head. Her corrected hare-lip corrugated into a tawny pucker.

"Go by Tweetie. Tweetie Droop."

"Okay, Tweetie Droop," I said. "Come meet Dore Tanner."

"He got him a funny name, ain't he?"

"That's right, he does. And my name's Lucien, but please call me Lu."

"Now you puttin' me on."

"Let me show you around, Tweetie," I said. I stopped at the hall closet to give her a box of latex gloves. I explained to her when to use them.

Tweetie crooked the box under one arm. "He married?" she asked.

"No," I said. "I'm Dore's partner."

"He got him a financee?"

"Ms. Droop," I tried again, hoping the use of her surname would sharpen her focus. "Let me explain. Dore and I are romantic partners. I love him very much. He is very ill with AIDS, a disease you can get through direct contact with the bodily fluids of an infected person. Use these gloves if you ever have to handle a bedpan or a throw-up basin. Have you ever worked with a person who has AIDS?"

"Know all about that," she frowned. "He got him a girl friend? Where his chirren?"

Bonnie joined us for supper after Tweetie had gone for the day.

"Face it, Dore. You're being tended by an idiot," I said.

"Oh, don't be so hard on yourself, Lu," you said, patting my hand.

Tweetie drove me slap crazy. I had to explain everything to her in excruciating detail. I would go over every item on our grocery lists and give her ample money. A half hour later, she would call from the store: "Got two bunches green onions. One got four fat ones, other seven thin ones." Ten minutes later: "Got lemon Clorox and regular."

"Ms. Droop: buy the one <u>you</u> prefer using."

"Tweetie," she said.

Tweetie was good to you. She bathed you and massaged your neuropathic back and feet with a cheerful willingness. After these sessions, you always smelled of

Chantilly, a pink body lotion for women Tweetie bought on one of her misguided missions to the store.

"So, how did you get the name 'Tweetie'?" I asked her one day.

"'Julia a purple name,' my Daddy always tell me after he divorce Momma. He call me 'Sweetie.' Said, 'Baby, I going to sweeten up that sour purple name what you Momma call you.' Over time 'Sweetie' become 'Tweetie.' When that happen, Daddy say, 'Tweetie give that heavy Julia name a lift.'"

"So, I not sweet no more?" I asked.

"'Yeah,' he say, 'you still sweet, but you growed up skinny and yellow like a bird too.' So 'Tweetie' stuck to me."

"Why did he think 'Julia" was a purple name?" you asked.

"I think it is too," I said.

"Then what color is my name?"

"You have to <u>ask</u>!? 'Dore' is golden, of course."

"And yours?"

"Bright silver, like moonlight. 'Lucien' means 'light.'"

"So do 'Lucifer,'" said Tweetie.

"So don't cross him, Tweetie," you said. "There's some holy water in the red cabinet by the bed when he starts drawing pentacles on the floor and lighting black candles."

"Now you puttin' me on," said Tweetie.

"What color is 'Bonnie'?" Bonnie asked.

"That a green name," Tweetie ventured.

"Deep-sea blue," I said. "Everybody knows that!"

The three of you looked at me, eyebrows raised.

"Now you puttin' me on," you said.

One morning ants appeared in a black mass on the kitchen counter after I had failed to rinse some late night ice cream bowls.

"Me and the ants be friendly like," Tweetie declared. "Leave 'em to me."

When I checked in later that afternoon, the ants had sent for reinforcements: squadrons trooped across the counter in thick convoy lines.

"I talked to 'em," Tweetie declared. "Stern-like. They be gone in three days. They moving outside with the honey I give 'em."

"Tweetie," I said, "these ants are moving in both directions, from outside in and inside out. Their fat queen has ordered a high feast for the entire ant hill right about now."

"Got us a agreement," Tweetie said. "You just give 'em some more honey in the morning."

I laced the honey with boric acid. The ants disappeared by the third day.

"See, Tweetie was right," you laughed.

"Dore! I poisoned them."

"You didn't!" you said.

"Good job, Tweetie," I said when she arrived before noon on the day the ants disappeared. "The ants are all gone in three days, just like you said. But in future, if you meet a cockroach, let me handle the negotiations."

"Never talk to 'em," she replied, shaking her head emphatically. "I squish 'em devil bugs!"

Tweetie stayed with us to the end. You were tolerant, often amused, always appreciative of her dim kindnesses. Bonnie winked at Tweetie's lapses and managed to coax the best out of her. We hired Tweetie to give the house a cleaning after we had wrenched our hearts out one Sunday afternoon sorting through your clothes.

When Bonnie gave her her final check, Tweetie wiped away two gold tears balled on her bronze cheeks. She took my hand: "It hard, him gone," she managed.

II

For cradle Catholics like you and me, the Church is background, culture, critical formation, perspective, at times antagonist. We live—and die—in its custom. Many of us still feel for the Church the regard we would maintain for a once loved mother now gone senile and sometimes vicious.

I called St. Philomene's the morning after you agreed to see a priest on the drive back from our last trip to San Francisco. A man picked up on the first ring. I decided to abbreviate but tell all so you would not have to ground the proposed visit.

"So, what's your address?" the man asked.

"When can the priest come?"

"How about now?"

Father Bill was not what we expected. In his late 40s, burly, he sported a grizzled beard and a mermaid tattoo on his forearm. He confessed to a weakness for Harleys, but arrived in a maroon sedan, a side panel spackled gray from an unsanded patch-up. A Roman collar topped a short-sleeved black shirt wisped with dog hairs.

I answered the door and ushered the priest into the family room. He trailed an odor of cigar smoke and antifreeze. You were sitting up.

"Can you excuse us for a moment?" Father Bill asked without looking back at me.

"There's a fresh pot of coffee on the counter," I said. I gathered the papers and closed myself in the study at the back of the house.

Nearly an hour elapsed. Suddenly I heard loud voices. I crumpled the paper section down in my lap and listened. Explosive laughter. Hooting. I opened the study door and walked down the hall. I peered into the family room.

"We forgot all about you!" you said.

"Come in! Come in!" Father Bill boomed as if he were hosting this little confab. Cookie crumbs joined the dog hairs on his black shirt.

The empty coffee pot was burning brown on the coffee-maker hot plate. Father Bill stayed until we offered him lunch: ex-Marine; widowed step-father of three children; recently ordained after a late calling heard one fall afternoon when his Harley had stalled on a back road in the orange hills; studying Spanish so he could minister to migrant farm workers up around Woodland. I tried a little Spanish out on him: he could not yet have ordered a taco at Taco Bell.

"I like him," you said. "He's easy to talk to."

I had just closed the front door behind him. We listened to his cracked muffler erupt, heard him sputter off down the street. I went out to sop up the oil slick I knew I would find on the driveway.

Father Bill returned for periodic visits over the remaining month and a half. He would officiate at your requiem mass. You had requested the old Marian hymn "Hail, Holy Queen Enthroned Above" as a post-funeral recessional from St. Philomene's.

"Why on earth did he want that old hymn to sing him out of church?" Father Bill asked.

I explained that gay men are often referred to as "Queens." "Hail, Holy Queen Enthroned Above" would refer to the post-mortem Dore. Get it?

"Let's have the organist play the melody," Father Bill laughed, "and we'll let the words resonate silently in our hearts."

TIDES

"I should go back to work," you would say. "I took disability too early." I would scan your meager face, thinking that you could not possibly live longer than a week or two at most if you did not eat more.

"If I stop breathing, do not try to revive me," you would insist. "Wait an hour and then call the funeral home." At that moment I was thinking that your color was creeping back, a faint rose-gold over the gray, that you had slept better the last few nights, that you had even tried a small green salad that afternoon along with a slice of chicken breast. Things were looking up.

We had no compass. We did not often talk about our course. You would pull through, rally. You were dying. The new pills seemed to be piquing your appetite. You did not think you could deal with much more. Your neuropathy was relenting at last. Your back hurt you less. The nausea attacks grew more frequent, more vicious. I coasted buoyant; I dropped sail, coded SOS, and looked for the life rafts. I hoped, despaired. You submitted to probing and weighing and dosing and doctor consulting, tried new medications, tried massages. I searched the horizon for rescue ships, for blue weather, for the low outline of an atoll.

But one anchor weighted all: a level of denial that allowed an odd sense of normalcy—illness and its undulations became stability and order. The daily tasks rolled in and out like the tides: the shopping and cooking and dishwashing, the laundry and the making of beds, the paper-reading and the bill-paying, the sitting beside you as we watched the evening news, hand in hand as if to front the day's catastrophes together. We could not fully comprehend what was happening to us. It was like looking at ocean luminescence in the dark: we saw clearly only by looking obliquely.

One evening in May, a little less than a month before you died, you wanted to read the papers in the living room after your attempts at eating a supper. You were chilly. You wanted a fire. Life for you had flattened out to such moments of comfort netted in the now.

I stacked the wood and laid the fire. You lay on the couch and watched with a critical eye. Then I sat on the floor by the side of the couch, holding the hand you dangled down to me.

"I could stay like this forever," I said in the wavering firelight.

"Within a half hour you'll be cramped and bored stiff."

You settled with a sigh into the pillows propped on the sofa arm as I moved to the chair across the room. You closed your eyes. The firelight dimmed and brightened, surged and ebbed. Your face rose in the flames. In the shadows, it receded. I watched you surface and submerge.

"What are you thinking?" you asked quietly from the firelit ebb and flow.

"A terrible thing is happening," I cried, fear drenching me like a breaker whitening over a reef. "A terrible, bitter thing."

A log settled. In the sudden light, you looked as if I had slammed across the room and slapped you hard.

BALANCE

"I think I understand it at last," I said, sitting on the side of the bed. "It came to me suddenly."

"Are you going to tell me?"

"I've lived close to fifty years now. I doubt I can be surprised anymore by life's sudden and arbitrary shifts between happiness and sadness. But I always thought happiness and sadness stood to each other as complete opposites, joy in one pan of life's scale, sorrow in the other pan. One pan teeters up, then life throws something into it, sending that pan down and the other pan up. Of course, we strive always to weight the joy pan more."

"And you see it differently now?"

"I got it wrong. Joy and sadness settle together in the same pan. They don't sort neatly into opposing pans at all. They seem inextricably bound together in life."

"So, what's in the other pan then?"

I faltered.

"I never believed in love before. You've made me a believer. And now I think that love fills the other pan. It increases the happiness of those fortunate enough to love. It soothes their sorrows. It makes the inevitable shifts between happiness and sorrow more manageable. At least loving you has done that for me."

You looked past me at a play of leaf shadow on the wall behind me.

"I have never been happier than since I loved you," I continued. "I have never been able to bear misfortune better."

You sighed. "Doesn't that place a burden on the one who is loved? He can't right all life's sadness for you. He may in fact cause sadness, like I'm doing to you."

"No, that's not it at all! The beloved need do nothing, only love in return."

I looked out at the darkening garden. A mockingbird trilled on a gray fencepost. I looked back at you. "So I can't let you go yet. Because then look what would be left: the empty pan."

Lowering my cheek to your chest, I heard there the balanced measure in my life at last.

THE ANATOMY OF GRIEF

"Welcome back!" I said when in bed with you after the surgical insertion of a PICC line in your upper chest to accommodate total parenteral nutrition. "To better times!"

"I hope so," you sighed. "But the idea of never tasting food again! Think of it!"

The next day a nurse came to review with me how to swab the port, flush the tubes, hook up the nutrients, start the feeding pump, stop it, disconnect the depleted bags, flush the tubes again, disinfect the port. He showed me what to do if the nutrients blocked in the tubes.

"This is what it sounds like if there's a problem," the nurse broke in. He set off the beeper.

"This is how to stop it," I said hurriedly. "I've done all this before," remembering Gary.

After I had hooked you up to the feeding pump for several sessions, your withering began slowly to reverse itself. A yellowish pink advanced up your throat, lapped onto your fallen cheeks, spilled over your gray lips. The daily feedings now energized you enough to rise from the couch to supervise a remodeling project you had begun: French doors in the family room to replace the slider, reparative tile work behind the stove. You were determined to leach vigor from the work bustle. Workmen whirled through the house; you napped through saws wailing and hammers banging. You joked with the workmen, poling the feeding bags swaying from the wheeled strut. You lurched through the quiet house inspecting the day's work. You began to shape solid again.

Tuesday evening, June 23

A little more than a week after you received the feeding tube, I slipped into a light sleep, attending to your breathing, not liking what I was hearing. You sipped air in shallow draughts. Too quickly cast it forth. Breath in short spasms. What did not come: a breath deeply taken. Skim-breathing. Goaded metronome. Rushed pendulum. Something was wrong.

I woke throughout the night to pace my breathing to yours, but I could not keep up. I needed to break your rhythm to inhale more deeply.

Wednesday morning, June 24

"I feel fine," you protested. "Don't bother the doctor."

The doctor listened to me in silence and then told me to pick up some prescriptions he would phone into the pharmacy by 3:00 P.M. You asked for sleeping pills. Your eyes darted at me when I emphasized <u>mild</u> sleeping pills, just a few to tide you over. In our early days together, you had left a copy of the Hemlock Society's *Final Exit* on the couch, your bookmark three-fourths through it. I murmured dismay and never saw the volume again.

I also asked for analgesics to relieve the pain in your right hip and lower back, your muscles now so wasted that they no longer cushioned the bone saddle centering you. I ordered ointment gauze patches to keep the bedsore Bonnie and I tended at the base of your spine from breaking open again.

The white pharmacy bag bulged with bottles and small boxes, including three squat vials bristling with red warnings, directions, counter-indications.

I took up the largest vial and read aloud its label: for pneumocystis carinii pneumonia. I glanced over at you in alarm: your eyes dashed at mine, searched them a moment, faltered away. If despair has a face it dares to show, then I saw it look through yours. This, you decided— and I feared—was endgame. Checkmate had come in a white pharmacy bag, winged on a hasty word.

I suspected you would play this out for only a few moves more to see if there was, by some miracle, a way out. But you knew. And I knew too: once past this, if that were possible, fresh horrors gaped their white obliterations.

You lay looking at the wall. My hand had fallen into my lap, as if the vial had been too heavy to bear. Neither of us said anything for a long time. But I could not give up. I would not let go.

I took your hand in mine. It lay there inert, with no play left in it, no pressure.

"We'll get through this too," I said. "Let's start the pills now."

I leaned across you to toss the pharmacy receipts into the bottom drawer of the red cabinet.

You pressed my hand hard. "Why bother, Lu?"

The pill regimen was complicated: multiple interacting meds to be administered at precise times and in various combinations, each pill particular in its requirements, a rout of exacting and unwelcome guests. I spent that evening lying next to you in bed, making up a meds chart for the next several weeks.

"It's just one more thing," I said. "Together we're stronger than this is, this new bastard."

You shrugged.

I tended to the bedsore: a puckered dormancy, its core mantled in new flesh nacreous as the skin of a pearl. I gave you pills, including a sleeping pill. I set the three clocks I had commandeered from other parts of the house, one for 1:00, one for 4:00, one for 7:00. I laid the different pill combinations adjacent to the clock signaling the hour each pile was to be taken.

In bed again, I massaged your hip and lower back. The pain raged there, refusing to vacate, a fractious lodger given to stomping and throwing itself against the walls.

I muddled awake each time an alarm sounded: one tinkled, one buzzed, one droned like a horsefly. When I awoke, I did not think I had really been asleep. You took the pills from me without speaking. You took one small sip of water for each pill because you could not hold your breath longer than a quick swallow: gulp, gasp.

You were directed to take the 4:00 meds with food. I coaxed you to sip milk thickened with yogurt, though this countered the doctor's prohibitions against dairy because of your persistent diarrhea. And you were no longer supposed to ingest food once on the feeding tube. Your body had become a fine-tuned betrayal, a disaster rigged up with trip-wires.

Thursday, June 25

Though cadenced, your breathing grew even more rapid, if possible, shallower. I waited until 8:00 to call the doctor, studying you, but before I could dial, his nurse rang to tell me she had made an appointment for you in radiology for chest x-rays. You groaned and shook your head no, but I was already laying out your clothes.

Before I helped you dress, I hoisted the cream-thick food bag from the refrigerator (it looked like regurgitated bird-pap, pre-digested for fledglings); warmed it; hooked it up; set the mechanism dials; listened for a soft churring, like insects droning in a night hedge; straightened the tubing now plumping with formula. In the car, you held the food bag and the power-pack mechanism like a befouled baby whose heavy diaper you did not want to change.

Once inside the clinic, fear frosted me as I gazed at you in the waiting room, a thin chrome rod now suspending the food bag over the wheelchair. No other patients there were as sick as you. Some soon would be. But you were dire. You hunched shrunken, collapsing in on yourself.

The first set of x-rays did not develop. I wheeled you in for a second set. We were told to wait to see if these could be scanned.

You begged me to take you home. You were dead tired, you panted, all done in. When I relayed this to a nurse at the front desk, she said to wait just a little longer. She did not look up from the notes she was writing in a patient file.

You pleaded with me to take you home. Now. NOW! I took your urgency back to the nurse, faith in these medical procedures still lingering. The nurse put her pen down. "I'll check on them for you," she said.

You were desperate. I think you were afraid they would hospitalize you. You may have feared dying in the waiting room. People looked at us, my head swaying back and forth trying to spot the nurse, your hand tensed on my forearm.

"Please!" you cried. "Please."

I wheeled you to the door. The nurse ran after us. "They're alright," she called down the parking lot. We never heard the results of the x-rays.

At home I got you undressed, put you into bed, gave you your 1:00 meds early so you could go right to sleep. Your eyes did not follow me around the room. They seemed to look inward, not focused. Tweetie arrived but backed out of the room when she saw I was there. You slept, but woke minutes later needing to go to the toilet, alarmed to find that you could no longer walk to the bathroom, even with my help. I brought you the bedpan. You had never had to use it before. You hoisted your hips up onto it, splaying clumsily in nakedness. You knew no dignity. Our eyes never met as I cleaned you with moist flush towels. I closed the bathroom door so you could not hear me retching as I rinsed the pan.

As soon as I came back into the room, you called for the basin.

"The basin? Are you sick?" I asked.

"The bedpan, the bedpan!"

You could no longer raise your hips onto its tilted rim. I slipped a blue chuck under you. "Just go on the chuck," I said. "I'll clean you."

A yellow froth curdled around your inner thighs.

I retched. It held me, my eyes clamped shut: "See what 'love' has led you to?" And I did see then the dread of it, its stern sadness, love's other face, just as I had earlier seen its wonder. I opened my eyes to see you gazing at me as if from far away.

"Call Tweetie. She knows what to do," you whispered. "You do not have to do this."

"I do!" I cried. "I do!"

239

"If I stop breathing, don't call anyone," you blurted, turning your face away from mine. "Just sit with me. Do not try to revive me."

"When it's your time, I promise to let it happen," I said. "But let's try. Stay with me a little longer."

As I cleaned you, you seemed to stare off unfocused through the water that had pooled at the sunken edges of your eyes.

Maple, your home-health-care nurse, arrived soon after.

"Mable?" I had asked on first meeting her.

"No, Maple. Like the syrup."

Anyone less syrupy than Maple could not be imagined. She looked like a don't-fuck-with-me attorney: hair cramped in a tight French twist, navy suit and paper-crisp white blouse, cool custodian of the feverish and infirm. She started when she entered the bedroom. She plied cuff and stethoscope, her brow smooth as a plate. She swabbed the port, checked the feeding tubes emerging from it. "Good job, Lu. You're hired!" she said cheerily.

"I have never seen anyone take such a sudden turn," Maple told me standing by her car. "Just Tuesday morning it all looked so promising. What happened?"

I felt as if I had let the enemy slip past to take the town, asleep at my post.

"He does not look good at all," Maple added, shaking her head. "You shouldn't wander too far from him this weekend. And if any of you have anything you need to tell him, tell it to him now. I'm having oxygen sent in."

A black heat swept up from the street asphalt.

Maple unbent as she saw me waver. She reached a hand out as if to steady me.

Shortly after 6:00, Ginny, your sister-in-law, arrived bearing red boxes of Chinese food for all of us. "Are you and Dore ready for a sunset ride in the convertible?" she warbled. "There's a container of egg flower soup when you return, Dore's favorite!"

"Dore's not doing well," I whispered. I did not need to say it. The atmosphere in the house—the hush, the brown shadows, the murmuring from your bedroom—told her enough. We left Ginny alone with you. After twenty minutes, she joined us in the family room, rimming a tissue under one eye.

Bonnie told us that you had questioned her about the pneumocystis. She had answered frankly—as she knew you expected her to—that your recovery would be long and taxing. You would have to fight with all your strength. We were all there to help with that. You nodded silently and looked away into the shadows.

The evening passed somehow. Ginny left for her hotel. Bonnie drifted out to her RV to read and smoke. We were alone.

"How are you doing?" I asked in that peculiar tone one uses with the sick, as if one's croon could be curative.

You shrugged. "Not well."

"Give the meds time," I said. "Do you feel bad?"

"Not good," you said.

You edged closer to me. The oxygen tubing hissed beneath your nose. You interrupted in odd places your sentences to snatch quick breaths.

"We've been together awhile now," you said, bringing my hand to your lips. "Not long enough, but such happy years!—amongst my happiest ever."

You had the grace to word even then what would make me happy and sad for years to come.

I checked the three clocks, sorted the pills over again, consulted the timetable I had drawn up. I filled the water cups.

"Do we have to tonight?" you asked. "I just want to sleep."

"We have to, yes!" I said.

"I'm so tired," you murmured.

I turned off the light. I heard you open the clasp of a leather pouch. You had been sleeping with your mother's ruby-glass rosary clutched in your hand for the last several nights.

Not more than an hour could have elapsed when you called my name. Something was wrong: I could hear it in your voice, a panic.

"There are people in the room!" you cried. "They're sitting in straight rows. They keep telling me to take my place, but I can't find a chair. They've hidden my rosary!"

I leaped from the bed and came over to your side. "I'm here," I said.

"But they're still in the room!" you cried. "Sitting in rows. They're telling me to sit down!"

I flipped on the lamp on the red cabinet. I knelt by the bedside. I turned your face so that our foreheads were touching.

"I'm here," I said. "It's just me here, no one else. You're in our bed safe with me, in our bedroom, like so many nights.

Your eyes still shot wide alarm.

"There's the dresser. There's the closet, the door leading to the bathroom. We're in the bedroom. There's no one else here but me," I said. "I'll keep you safe."

You brought your hand to my cheek as if to realize me.

"And your rosary has fallen into the bedclothes." I put the beads in your hand and closed your fingers over them.

Your face slowly softened. "You're my savior!" you panted.

I watched you until the one o'clock alarm sounded. I gave you the pills. You slept. I turned off the lights. I went back to my side of the bed.

"Watcha fixin'?" you asked in that singing tone you always greeted me with on entering the kitchen, my back to you as I prepared dinner. I shot awake in the dark. You repeated the question.

I raised myself on an elbow, put my hand on your chest. "Dore," I said, low, calm. "We're in bed. It's nighttime. I think you're dreaming. I'll stay up with you until you sleep."

You turned towards me. I heard you sigh, settle, snore lightly.

I could tell it was 4:00 by the drone of that particular alarm clock. You refused the milk mixture. You choked on the pills, unable to get them down.

What seemed like only moments after we had settled again, I heard the covers thrashing. You sat up. "We're late!" you said. "We need to leave for your sister's. She's having us over for dinner." You dropped one leg over the bedside. I hurried over to your side of the bed, restrained you from rising.

243

"No," I said. "Mary and Joe are in Louisiana. We were at her house at Christmas. It's just a dream."

You lowered yourself slowly into the bed again, frowned at me doubtfully. "What's happening to me?" you asked.

Friday, June 26

I lay with you until I was certain you slept soundly. Then I crept out of bed, went out of the room, and shut the door. I stood in the doorway of the study, Bonnie's back to me.

"He's dying," I said.

Bonnie clenched but did not turn around. Then she stood, shut down the computer. Still she did not say anything.

"He's off and on in dementia," I added. "He's been hallucinating throughout the night. He's found it difficult to come out of the delusions. I've been calling it 'dreaming,' but he knows what it is. He will not put up with this."

"Why don't you go home and rest?" Bonnie said. "I'll sit with him."

"I'll be back around 2:00," I said. I went to my house and fell asleep on the couch. I could not bring myself to sleep alone in my bed.

I returned to you at 1:30. Tweetie had sponge-bathed you and dressed you in a pair of aqua pouch-fronted gym shorts, at one time ripe and sexy on you. Now you reminded me of those saggy old men who parade around in these shorts at San Francisco's Folsom Street Fair long after they should not be seen in them. Tweetie had gotten you into a red-plaid flannel pajama shirt against the chill of the air conditioner, thereby shattering a lifetime of careful good taste in your clothing. Past all that now.

Bonnie had caught me up on the morning. Soon after I left, you had tried to rise from bed to get ready for work. You were bewildered by the oxygen regulator under your nose, the feeding tube, the condom-catheter collecting your dark brown urine. When Bonnie restrained you, you had returned immediately to yourself.

"I'm in dementia?" you asked.

"Drifting at times," Bonnie explained it. All incidents of dementia ended at this point.

Bonnie had described to your doctor this new turn you had taken. He ordered morphine patches. You asked me to go with Ginny to pick them up at the pharmacy.

"Why do you want us both to go?" I asked.

"Ginny doesn't know the way to the pharmacy. The patches are expensive. She can put them on her credit card until my insurance covers them."

I looked at you doubtfully.

We were away for less than an hour. Bonnie was sitting on the front steps smoking a cigarette when we drove up.

"He wants to see each of you alone," she said as we approached the house. "He wants to say goodbye."

I was afraid. I knew that whatever you worded, whatever I said, I would hear over and over for the rest of my life.

We gathered around the bed. Bonnie applied a morphine patch at your left breast.

"Two of them," you demanded.

They left you and me alone together.

"I can't do this anymore," you said. "I need to go now. Let me go, okay?"

I nodded.

"Let me go."

I leaned over to kiss you, but you put a hand up on my chest to stay me.

"Let me go, Lu."

"Yes," I got out. You seemed to need to hear the words. "It's your time. I know it too now."

"Help Joe and Bonnie," you said.

"Be there for me on the other side," I blurted. "I won't be afraid if you're there to help me over." Cliches crowd up when the mind fails one.

"As soon as you lift the latch, you'll see me."

I tried to smile.

"Help Joe and Bonnie," you repeated. You squeezed my hand. "Tell Ginny to come in."

I went to sit with Bonnie on the front steps.

"He wants to bring it to a close himself. That's why he got me and Ginny out of the house. He has a plan."

"Yes," Bonnie said.

"No," I cried. "You can't help him."

Bonnie looked at me wearily, drew on her cigarette. "I'm not going to deny him anything right now," she said. "I'm not going to tell him what to do."

"I'm going to plead with him not to do this."

"Fair enough," Bonnie said. "I'm not going to tell you what to do either."

Ginny came out, blotting her eyes. "He wants you and Joe, Bonnie. He thinks Lu and I should stay in the family room together for a while."

"They're going to kill him," Ginny whispered to me as we sat together.

I went into the bedroom. Bonnie was sitting in the chair beside the red cabinet. Joe sat up next to you in my place on the bed. Bonnie wore latex gloves to avoid leaving fingerprints should any inquiries be made. She was unwrapping syringes she had laid out on the red cabinet. You were propped up in bed. You were drawing liquid Percocet into the syringes, an amber opiod liquid you had poured into the kidney-shaped basin.

"Dore," I said. "There's another way. I'll get you hooked up to a morphine drip. We'll see that you sleep through it."

You did not pause in your work.

"I've never asked for anything from you," I cried. "But I'm asking for something now: Do not do this."

"I cannot give this to you," you said.

"But what if you don't succeed? What if you hurt yourself and make things worse? Then we would have to call someone in. Or have you taken to the hospital. There would be inquiries."

"I'll succeed." You filled another syringe and handed it to Joe. A shopping bag of unfinished prescriptions you had hoarded for just this purpose propped itself against your thigh. You had poured the new sleeping pills into a pile on top of the red cabinet.

"Do this one thing for me. Let me call the doctor. The morphine drip will be kinder and just as sure."

You paused. None of us moved. A filled syringe was poised in your hand, your pajama shirt opened to the PICC line port above your heart. I knew that your next word would announce the way it would be.

"Please!" I cried. "Let me get you the morphine drip. It will be easier on you. We can take it from there."

You lowered the syringe. "I'll give you an hour."

I dialed the clinic number I knew by heart. Another doctor was on weekend call, but your doctor had told her you were failing.

"I need you to send someone out right away to hook Dore up to a morphine drip," I said.

"We sent morphine patches out this afternoon," she said. "Is he using one?"

"Two," I said, "but he's planning to bring it to an end himself."

"Does he have the means?"

"He's going to inject himself with Percocet."

"Percocet is a pill."

"He has liquid Percocet left over from when he had the PICC line inserted into his chest. He's already filled several of the large syringes I use to flush his feeding tube. He's going to inject himself through the port. He has also counted out a pile of sleeping pills and pain medications from past prescriptions."

"Oh," she said, "that'll hurt him. Tell him to wait. I'll send someone out."

I went back into the bedroom. "The morphine drip is on its way."

You looked up at me with a studied expression, then looked away. What passed between us in that long gaze? I had wrested your death away from you. I had no choice: Death by your own hand would have thrown me into a grief so deep that I do not think I could have climbed out of it. But what did your concession cost you, this tossing your last card into the box, pulled from hiding under a haunch, from behind your back? You long endured the virus's ruthless victory. Everywhere it won, all medical barricades quickly swept aside, card after card dealt into the box. You had at last made a stand: in a single act you would decide your own fate, wrest control at last. You would command the field. You would spite the virus. You would have your way.

This was your last card, and I had pleaded with you not to play it. Now you were throwing it into the discard box with all the other cards you had had to give up. You had arrived at the place where Carl and Roger, Sean, Gordon, Corey and Jeff, Gary, Laird, Zach and Ben and Jake had arrived before you: all the cards had now been given up. Your hand was empty. My training exercise was supposed to have prepared me for this moment. It had not prepared me to recognize that I had had to throw all my cards in as well, my desperate hopes that you would be spared, that the new medicines would work, that I could hold on to you for years more.

Bonnie leaned back in the chair and snapped her gloves off. Joe scooped the pills up and carried the filled syringes out of your reach. What did it take for you to see those syringes hastened away, the sack of leftover meds, death in a grocery bag, disappear out of harm's way after having planned this for so long? Was this your last defeat? And your last gift to me?

I called Father Bill, the priest from St. Philomene's, but he was on retreat in Chico for the weekend. I phoned the chaplain on call at Mercy Hospital. He arrived, a bald, angular stranger, slim as a stoat. He heard your confession after we left the room, then called us in for your anointing. Then the priest left, a hand lingering on your shoulder.

A nurse from hospice passed him in the hall. She carried a black satchel, her tight curls purple in the light of the lamp on the red cabinet. She took your vital signs frowning, her eyes gliding impassively around the anxious faces in the room. She started the morphine drip. The administering mechanism could be pressed, though supposedly regulated to prevent an overdose. "You need only press it every fifteen minutes or so, as needed. With two morphine patches already on, you could give him too much otherwise," she cautioned. "And I'd retain the oxygen: it'll make him more comfortable, especially with his struggle with pneumonia."

"And the feeding machine?" I asked.

"If you disconnect it abruptly, it will more than likely throw his system into shock," she said. "I'm not sure he could take that."

I met your gaze.

The nurse saw. She whispered to me: "I won't tell you what to do. He has the right to refuse any further treatment, including the feeding tube." Then she cupped my arm at the elbow and leaned close: "I'm on duty until 8:00 in the morning. Call me if you need anything." She pressed her card into my hand.

Bonnie picked up the mechanism to release the morphine. She pressed it repeatedly from that point on.

Your eyes glazed, then closed.

I gathered the basin, the saline solution, new flushing syringes. You opened your eyes and nodded. Here was our careful passing you out of our care. I unhooked, flushed, folded the feeding tube. Bonnie pressed the morphine regulator again and again.

Your eyes fluttered closed. When I kissed you, your lips gathered, slowly straightened. I lay down next to you. I brushed the hair off your forehead, laid my face in the join of your neck and shoulder. I heard Bonnie press the morphine regulator again, again.

Then—suddenly—I heard a long, clotted inhalation, like a wave rolling rocks; then a high, thin, sorrowful sigh. I raised my head. Bonnie's hand was suspended over the morphine regulator. We stared at each other. And the rough inhalation grated again, a peak pause, then the slow expiration, its high, long sigh sorrow given voice.

A grief rose so welling that it overwhelmed reason: "I hurt you. I caused this. It would have been over by now if I had not interfered, if I had let you have your way." I listened, breathless, to your farewell to a world you had loved and were leaving too soon. I had been told that this last breathing, this death rattle, does not denote pain, only a final letting go, a giving up, throat muscles gone slack. Still, Death fought hard and dirty.

"Let it be over! Let it be over!" I prayed in a despairing mantra. Bonnie pressed more morphine.

Suddenly the ragged breathing stopped. I raised myself on one arm. Your breathing went shallow and regular. We signaled those waiting in the other room. When they had gathered, you opened your eyes, gazed slowly around the room, and then at me. You had been breathing through your mouth, your lips now white and cracked.

"Would you like some water?" I whispered.

You made as if to shake your head no, but then your eyes rolled back. I could see nothing but white, a blanking out of that blue wonder of you. You closed your eyes again for the last time. The gentle, regular breathing continued for another few moments. You took three short, gulping breaths. Your breathing stopped. A soft suss drifted through your open lips. Then all was still. The three clocks on the red cabinet showed 5:27 A.M. on Saturday, June 27.

Sunrise.

"You did it right," I whispered in your ear. "You did everything right. Go safely now."

There was weeping in the room. I did not look up. Soon I was alone with you. I think I slept. Then I lay looking at you, at the you not you anymore, at the still you. Your eyes, your mouth were closed, your face set.

I needed lessons in how to relate to your dead body. This was like a first date. I could now look long at you without causing you discomfort, but I kept looking away, at your hair, which I smoothed, at the elegant careless curl of your fingers, which I closed in mine, your nails clouding a deep purple at the cuticles.

Your dead body shocked me in its beauty and vacancy. You had fought the virus: now you looked the victor uninterested in the prize—serene, unscarred, your face more blank than peaceful. Your body lay tight and discarded, a beautiful surface for morning light to shimmer over with wing-shadow and leaf-play through the drawn shades.

I angled your face towards mine, our foreheads touching. I closed my eyes and lay there with you I do not know how long.

No transcendence. No meaning. Nothing. Just an absence, an empty husk of love and loss.

Bonnie came into the room. "Come join the living," she said gently. "The nurse will be here soon, then the funeral home people."

"A minute longer," I said without moving. I took you full in my arms. I let my hands contour your body.

I looked at you a last time from the bedroom doorway. You had prohibited the gaze of mourners. You would lie unembalmed in a closed wooden casket. I did not want to see you touched by strangers or rolled from our bedroom strapped onto a gurney, zippered into a body bag. They would wheel you through the new French doors, the only time you would ever cross through them. I kissed you one last time before leaving. You were still warm.

You died in 1998. Since 1996, many teetering on death's jagged brink had been summoned to life again in dramatic reversals brought about by the same new synergistic combinant therapies you were taking. These miracle drugs did not work for you: you did not draw the golden ticket; you did not win the AIDS lottery.

Your doctor explained to me, post-mortem, that early on you had been given large doses of AZT, the first real AIDS drug, a white pill banded in blue with a unicorn prancing over the name of the pharmaceutical company—WELLCOME—that had profited outrageously from those desperate for the pill.

AZT's impact was often dramatic in the short run, especially in the high doses you were taking every four hours as signaled by a beeper, but AZT prompted the virus to mutate within weeks. In addition, AZT was toxic to bone marrow, causing serious depletions of red or white blood cells and too often leading to the development of various lymphomas. Your doctors had followed AZT with a slew of other newly developed drugs, most also taken in isolation, before it dawned on researchers that interactive combinations of these drugs might prove more effective than monotherapies. So, by 1998, your HIV virus was resistant to the drugs now being taken in combinations that worked. The assault on your body of all the noxious drugs you had been taking was so extreme that you could not recover from the physical wreckage these drugs had abetted the virus in reducing you to. And you were by then apparently too weak to take prophylactic bactrim against the PCP that finally ended your life. Others more fortunate than you on the new combinant therapies were exhilarated at their soaring T-cell counts and dramatic plunges in HIV viral loads.

You died in the midst of new hope and widespread elation and relief—too late to board the festive cruise ship ferrying so many stricken with advanced AIDS to jubilant new lives. You were not able to attend the party, an added grief to us who wanted so desperately to join the celebration, the Eastering of so many we had given up for dead.

According to amfAR (The American Foundation for AIDS Research), 410,800 Americans and millions worldwide had died of AIDS from 1981 to 1998. amfAR logged 20,108 AIDS deaths in the United States during 1998 alone. You were one of them. I joined a multitude left to mourn.

At my house after leaving you that final time, I choked on two of your sleeping pills, forced myself dry-eyed into my white bed, curled into a hollow crescent away from your picture on the nightstand, faced the wall.

POSTMORTEM

Did grief begin with your pacing the night rooms in throat pain, unable to eat, unable to sleep, each swallow a stabbing? Did it begin with my hearing that you would lose your hair during chemotherapy? Or when you, brittle and yellow as old newspaper, entered the hospital just before that last Thanksgiving? Did grief begin in the cloying, deodorized darkness of that hotel room in Tahoe when you sobbed your heart out in my arms? Or when I wheeled you in the chair away from your April farewell luncheon with your office colleagues after you had wrenched yourself away from the career you loved?

Was there ever time for grief in our alternations of hope and denial, the rallying and the sad reversals, during the distractions of dailiness evidenced in the black-lacquered drawers in your red cabinet of all lost things, all the things to get done, the mail and bill paying, the relentless doctor appointments, the loitering in pharmacies waiting for prescriptions to be filled, the grocery shopping, the many memorial services for friends, vacuuming, making beds, washing clothes, meal preparations, eating— or your trying to eat—those endless television cooking shows you stared at some pathetic substitute for your lost hunger?

When did I begin to grieve? After the three short final breaths silencing those grating inhalations, those long sighs? Grief was there then, but it did not begin then. It is just that when everything else was over, grief was all that was left.

PART IV: REGAINING EQUILIBRIUM

When do our senses know anything so utterly as when we lack it? . . . For to wish for a hand on one's hair is all but to feel it. So whatever we may lose, very craving gives it back to us again. Though we dream and hardly know it, longing, like an angel, fosters us, smooths our hair, and brings us wild strawberries.

--Marilynne Robinson, *Housekeeping*

AFTERMATH

I

At your funeral, the last three rows of St. Philomene's were filled with gaunt clients of the AIDS Foundation, Rhetta Sproul and other caseworkers, and assorted volunteers who had come to mourn with me, a tragic chorus among whom I had myself so often numbered.

Two days later, I boarded a plane for a week in San Diego where I worked several times a year scoring papers. The nights were mine to do as I liked: I had a rental car, a hotel room, a reputation to maintain in the bars.

I diffused through finality and closure, muffled in relief that your suffering in those mortal days was over now. Throughout the ritual rounds of the funeral days, I sank into conclusion, like the numb seepage of serum after a blow, before the mind can register pain or record, in alarm and outrage, the damage. How could I be in shock after an outcome so expected? I had seen the hammer falling in slow motion. How could I be stunned?

The hour and a half flight from Sacramento south was a motionless hanging in air, a strange stasis under a sky blue and hard as a marble. I have seen the sunlight in the south of France. The shadows weight blue-black there; colors float with startling intensity. The light in San Diego is similar, as it is in Palm Springs. As I walked out of that white airport, my eyes dazzled. The palm trees exploded, each green fan edged in silver.

Where were you in all of this? I do not know. I summoned you in memory all during the week, and you came, at least the feel of you did. My heart was oddly untroubled by vacancy. I concluded you had found your way. You were free, and I was too.

This sufficient heart proved temporary.

I sat in bars every night after reading papers all day, was rarely alone in my hotel room. I found comfort in the lusty, breathing bodies of men, commingled again with the living. I had held your dead body close. I now recoiled from death, from its shocking intimacy. My body found solace in arms that could embrace me, in bodies ripe with the pulse and thrust of life.

Juan made me forget you, propped up on the bathroom counter at a perfect coital height. "What happened to you?" the Chief Reader asked the morning after Rick had fucked me roughly, the cut over my right eye the result of a scrape from the cast on his left wrist as he pulled my head back for a bruising kiss. I topped a young sailor I met at the San Diego baths, just off-ship, randy and rompingly calisthenic after a lonely four-month tour.

My body denied your still body. It disclaimed death. Guilt? None at all.

I first met Javier at this reading in San Diego the year before. He taught English in the Honors Program in a San Diego high school. He came from a family of undocumented migrant workers following ripening crops from California to Michigan and back again, sleeping in rusting trailers and unpainted sheds stifling in summer heat redolent of cow urine. He had earned a scholarship to Stanford, prompted to apply by a counselor at one of the seven high schools he drifted among.

Javier invited me to go with him to the top of the Park Manor Hotel in Hillcrest to ogle the men at the Friday evening crush. Surveying a ballroom crammed with men, some of such beauty as to turn the heart hollow, I shouted in Javier's ear: "With so many to choose from every Friday night, how can you still be single?"

Javier motioned me outside to a gallery running along the eighth floor to a patio thronged with men. We stood looking out over downtown at jets needling their flightways between tall buildings, at the distant lights of Tijuana on the hill over the border.

"I lost my lover to AIDS four years ago," Javier said. "We lived in San Francisco for six years before he died. After I was alone, I moved back here to be closer to friends. I just can't get over losing Cruz."

"Four years is a long time," I said.

"Have you ever lost a lover?" he asked.

I did not want to talk about you in this throng of living men, but I could not then deny you, even here.

"My lover died just over a week ago," I said at last.

Javier pivoted slowly to me, not just his head, his whole body. "A week?" he whispered.

"I'm doing alright," I said quickly. "I needed to get away. His death was the conclusion of a long illness."

"AIDS, right?"

I nodded. Javier looked away, out over the great darkness of Balboa Park. "You'll see," he said.

II

I flew back to Sacramento on the day of my fiftieth birthday. Bonnie picked me up at the airport and took me out to dinner to mark the event. She invited Melanie. I threw back two martinis at the bar before we were seated at a table. I was animated, still glowing from the excesses of San Diego. After dinner, two waiters approached with a small carrot cake sputtering with a single white candle.

"How kind of you to minimize the blaze," I murmured.

The waiters sang "Happy Birthday." I blew out the candle, and then my face warped into what must have been a ghastly smile. The waiters glanced briefly at each other, faltered, backed away.

Your family waited until I returned from San Diego to sort your clothes and to go through your possessions. We started in the kitchen, then tackled the Christmas ornaments. Box after box of them filled the upper half of the hall closet. You collected ornaments year round. You had to enter Christmas shops wherever you found them, whatever the season. I would wait on the sidewalk until you emerged toting a small bag, smiling furtively, as if you had just scored big from a drug dealer in south Sacramento.

We finished for the day and had cocktails. Your brothers drifted off to bed after supper, leaving Bonnie and me to talk outside in the warm summer night.

"How are you doing?" she asked, feeling her way warily.

"I think fine," I said.

"Is it difficult for you to go through Dore's things?"

"They're just things. We used them in living. They don't mean anything to me."

"I want you to choose a couple of things that <u>would</u> mean something to you," she said.

"I don't need that," I said.

"You know he loved you, right?"

I nodded. We sat in silence for a while longer. I stood to go.

"Come back tomorrow, if you can," Bonnie said. "And think about what you'd like."

I asked Bonnie for the red lacquer cabinet by your bedside and the picture of the two of us in the cream and lavender desert that rested on it.

"Take them," Bonnie said immediately. "But why that beat-up old thing? Frankly, we'd tagged it for a Goodwill pick up. I thought you might want something more personal. Would you wear his jade ring?"

III

The next morning we sorted through your travel slides. In the afternoon we would go through your clothes.

You had wandered the world with a restless hunger, as if you had had a premonition that you would soon lie still in a dark, narrow place. You took hundreds of slides and slotted them into carousels ready for the projector. Like a diligent accountant, you placed and dated the carousel boxes. We clicked the earliest carousel into the projector.

You materialized on the wall nearly life-sized, very young, straps from a backpack banding your chest like parentheses. You looked as if you were going away to summer camp. Someone had snapped you at the airport.

The room was silent. Dust motes rioted in the light beam. And then you were gone. The projector clicked to the next image, fields of sunflowers against a gray sky, apparently shot through a rain- streaked train window. In France, according to the carousel box.

I grew eager for your image, scanned each slide for a glimpse of you. The slides revealed a fascination with church spires and steeples, glimpses of them and from them, oblique views which you had apparently taken while lying on your back in some pigeon-spattered square, cityscapes framed by gargoyles or rude Gothic carvings. Then more landscapes.

"We'll never get through all these," Joe said.

"There's a manual clicker," Bonnie said. "You take it, Lu."

I rushed us through France. Image after image flashed, whirred into focus, faded. And then there you were again, standing outside an *auberge*, frowning into the sun, my thumb arrested on the advance that would send you into the darkness again.

The slide box was dated 1972. You would have been 23. You were a bit shlubby, a bit untidy. I would not have recognized you. The body I knew was big-boned but keen as an oar. Here you looked soft, your hair sticking up in clumps as if you had not washed it for several days. You looked sad, tentative. Lonely. Like an exile wanting to return home. Through a trick of light, you seemed to look directly at me.

I handed the remote to Bonnie. She let your image linger a moment, then sent you back into the darkness.

"There are a lot of slides," Tom yawned.

Bonnie began to click through the slides more rapidly. We journeyed throughout Europe, into Egypt, Morocco, the Middle East. I saw you gripping the belled reins of a camel, looking down mistrustfully at a dark handler flashing white, crooked teeth. We had yet to progress through southern Africa, Australia and New Zealand, parts of Asia as indicated on the slide boxes. Whenever, rarely, you materialized on the wall, Bonnie paused. I saw you through all the years I did not know you. I learned your clothes, hairstyles, body shapes. What did not waver was the look of the exile.

You were nowhere near out of the closet back then, occasionally larking through gay bars in Sacramento and tramping through the baths in San Francisco looking for tricks, sometimes booking gay cruises, gathering with other men loping through life mateless, packing together in rutting season, bodies honed and toned in gyms and spas, clean depilatoried.

All gay men of our generation are exiles, displaced persons, especially gay men still locked in their closets. We are refugees, never, in the deepest part of ourselves, feeling that we really belong in straight society. And we are haunted by our separateness in ways that straight people who love us or work with us can never know. Our exile, however, prompts our paradoxical exhilaration in being sexual outlaws, on the run and unencumbered. Freedom, a rootedness deep in selfhood, our marginality, our liminal positioning in the world, the queer double vision: these flash in us a heady exuberance, though tempered by our displacement.

I knew that gay look in your eyes. In you I could spy myself, all the sadness we could not show during those closeted years. No one in the straight world could see it, or was expected to look for it. You and I were solo voyagers on different vectors, whose fortunate windways converged one accidental November night not so long ago.

You were on the wall again, in the Chianti Hills above Florence, sunset over the distant Arno, the Giotto tower a red-gold finger pointing into a gilded blue. You gazed steadily into the camera. You did not smile.

"He always looks a little sad," said Bonnie. A lesbian, she noticed this too.

"I don't see that," said Tom.

"Neither me," Joe said. "He's just not smiling there."

IV

Things got worse.

We decided we had better start to sort your clothes. We could finish the slides later. Soon your bed was covered in divided heaps: starched, folded shirts were stacked like sheets of paper; balled up socks tumbled among piles of underwear; belts slithered from under folded trousers. We emptied the closets, all the drawers.

"I have to go," I said.

"Stay for dinner," Bonnie urged.

I could not say anything.

Bonnie put her hand on my shoulder and peered into my eyes. "Let's talk soon," she said. "Just you and me."

I drove home. I piled the clothes they insisted I take on my bed in a tangle. I burrowed among them and lay, dry-eyed, watching the light fade in the room. I nestled my cheek into the folds of your robe all night. It smelled of you.

V

Things got worse.

I started to need to talk about you. The only person I could talk with was Bonnie. I exhausted her. At times she interrupted my monologues, not because they pained her—she needed to talk too—but because they looped in dull rounds like a serpent searching for its tail.

I found my way to your house every evening. I sipped martinis. Bonnie drank warm Tab from the can and smoked cigarettes. We sat outside watching darkness settle over the redwoods and stars blink on.

The need to talk was urgent, a junkie's habit. I was trying to fix you. I thought to shape you in syllables, to rescue you from suspension.

Memory daubed like a Cubist: it collaged scenes from many odd angles all at once, shaded in strange chromatics. Some nights, memory turned ventriloquist: it amplified conversations and mouthed novel dialogue, not bothering to disguise its moving lips. It snapped pictures like a daft photographer, fiddling with exposures and overlaying images. I talked and talked, desperate to make memory stand still.

Bonnie would say, "I remember that differently." I would hotly contest. She would draw on her cigarette, regard me coolly with a narrowed eye, her head tilted. "We simply saw it from different perspectives," she would say, puzzled at my insistence on having you my way.

I talked to exonerate myself. Crickets coded in the star jasmine as I pleaded: Did I do everything I could for you? Did you fight hard enough?

"He did it right," said Bonnie, "and you helped him."

Talk and talk. Therapy on the cheap. Your dying, my helpless loving you had shattered the neat, poised, safe life I had lived for fifty years. Here now jabbered a lost coherence. I shuffled a clutter of fractured gestalts: love may be real, but it could neither protect nor exalt, so what good was it? The best endured the worst cataclysms. The world was never schemed in mercy. You would be forgotten. When I died, both of us would be digested in the yellow bile of Time.

As these evenings went on, night after night, I saw in Bonnie's eyes the slow gather of alarm. She concluded I needed a help beyond her. I did. I just could not make my life, your death come clear. Words funneled up like shredded paper in a dust devil.

VI

Things got worse.

I noticed one day in the paper that a local hospital was convening a grieving group as part of its social outreach services to the community. The ad specifically solicited participants who had lost someone to AIDS, but did not exclude anyone else.

"Is it a gay group?" Bonnie asked.

"I don't think so," I said. "At least not exclusively."

"That may matter," Bonnie said.

It did matter.

I had a preliminary interview with the therapist. He was gay. He seemed defensive, possibly degree conscious. I regretted giving him my business card on introducing myself.

"By the way," he asked as I stood to leave, "how long were you with your late partner?"

"Several years," I said.

"Not very long!" He raised his eyebrows.

He should have known that gay men in the era of AIDS often had to become masters of short intensity, that whole emotional lives could be fused into a density that would take years to penetrate.

Eight of us gathered at the first meeting. The session began with "check-ins," chronicles of what had brought us to the group. Kevin, an acquaintance of mine, was there after losing his lover three months before in a grim battle with Hepatitis C, abetted by HIV, the lover having turned yellow as an Easter chick during his last days. Kevin began these weekly check-ins with a breathy blubbering. Then he talked: he had had to quit his job after his lover died, the very thing he should never have done, I thought.

The wife of a dentist had called it quits several months before after a gruesome struggle with breast cancer, leaving him at 42 with two children, now seven and ten. He looked down at his hands when he talked about how needy his children always seemed to be, how they did not like staying with their aunt. Flat affect.

One woman had lost her father the year before. He had squinched his face up into a startled question and keeled over the barbecue while flipping burgers outside. She was there to figure out why she felt no grief whatsoever. Never had

Three women from the suburbs I judged to be therapy junkies. They had been together in grieving groups before. They enjoyed their time there because they had an audience. One of these women was dealing with the loss of her best friend's six-year-old daughter to leukemia two years before, apparently haunted by a little crone-face staring up from a white bed at St. Jude's; another to the recent death of an elderly neighbor she had grown up living next to but had not seen in years; the third to the recent death of a distant cousin in an auto crash in upstate

New York. I dubbed these minor cases. I became adjudicator of grief. I knew this was wrong. So I took on guilt.

My turn: I said after losing you I could not right myself, could not make things come together and cohere, somehow could not mold my life again and live it. I could not look at anyone in the group.

"Oh, tell me about it!" started up a fleshy young blonde woman named Rachel before I had finished. "I have trouble even getting up off the couch. I just lay there all day flipping TV channels. My three brats start whining, 'Get up, Mommy. Let's go to the store. We're hungry.' I can't take it. I just flop over and tell them shut up. Some days I can't even get them dressed to go to school and they just sit around bugging me. Since my momma died three months ago, I can't call nobody to cut me a check when my welfare runs out at the end of the month. I couldn't hardly scrape up bus fare to get me out here this evening 'cause no one would give me a ride."

"I think you and your children need a lot more help than this grieving group can give you," I erupted when she paused. A silence fell on the room. The therapist looked at me a long time, then flicked his face away.

Before the next session, we were assigned to write a letter to the person we were grieving, expressing our anger with them for leaving us. Predictable. So Kubler-Ross. . . .

I kept a copy of what I wrote:

Dore: In middle life I find myself lost in a dark wood. I feel Dante's opening lines of *The Divine Comedy* for the first time now. I spend my nights piecing our time together in words. You would feel sorry for Bonnie as she slogs through my word spew. But if I can only say it all and get

270

the words right, I can keep you. I can make sense of it all. I'm supposed to be angry with you. That's a crock: You did not want to leave until forced to. You fought hard, but death won. And how can I be angry with fate and chance? That's like slapping the sea or stabbing the sky. I cannot even imagine myself angry with you.

"I did write the letter," I said when it came my turn in session, "but I just cannot read it tonight."

"Part of your problem," said Rachel with the unfed kids, "is that you ain't got God in your life. Everybody needs God, even those who think they don't. Can't go it alone! I don't know where I'd be without God and the Harvest Church out in Roseville."

"Worse off than you are?" was forming like a sour curd on my tongue, but one of the therapy dipsos headed me off: "Sounds like denial to me. You don't get better by bottling it up like you do. Anger is one of the necessary stages of grieving. If you can't talk about it, maybe you should try to get it all out in private by writing some waaa-waaa book nobody'll ever read."

So here is the book.

Comments on my silences became a refrain in future sessions: "You sit here and hardly ever say anything to us, even in check-ins," complained the woman whose cousin had crashed in upstate New York. "How are you going to get any help from us?"

I looked down at my hands. "You're right," I spat.

"He's entitled to feel whatever he feels," said the therapist at last, "and he can talk or not talk, whatever he wants."

I developed a bad attitude.

Why did I continue to attend, week after dismal week? Two reasons: First, I did feel better trying to address my emptiness with action. Doing something, anything, even this, felt better than crumpling dry-eyed in bed wrapped in your robe. Also, Kevin and I would go for a cheap dinner at the same Mexican taqueria after every meeting. He cried over the chips and salsa. I watched with envy his fat tears. I would go home afterwards and try to force myself to cry—like sticking my fingers down my throat to vomit when I had drunk too much.

What I came to realize was the nature of grief: It is not soft. It is not gentle. Melancholy and grief have nothing in common. Grief is not nostalgia. It is a cold, dark cell with obdurate blank walls, echoing within and paralyzing, with a trap door locked from outside. Once inside, no outside voices ever really penetrate. It is the loneliest place I have ever been in.

The grieving group disbanded the week before Thanksgiving, in time to prepare us for the onset of a holiday season bereft. The farewell potluck was a meager spread of church-lady food. I brought a cheesecake and watched the young woman with the hungry kids slide a couple of pieces down. I sent the rest home with her. The dentist said we would keep in touch for sure though neither of us had any intention of ever doing so. Kevin cried as he told me about this guy he had just met who worked at the bottle recycling center behind the Safeway: "I think it's love, Lu!" I sucked green jello salad from my teeth as the three therapy junkies pressed each other in tearful embraces and hinted at another group forming early in the new year.

VII

Things got worse.

During the next weeks, Christmas coiled into swags and wreaths. I went to a round of dinners and parties. People were careful of me, though one of my friends complained that I was not much fun to be around these days. "Shape up!" he said. "This is so unlike you!" Oh, did that ever help.

I made plans to fly home to Louisiana the Monday preceding Christmas. The Sunday noon before my departure, I attended a Christmas luncheon for the clients and volunteers of the Sacramento AIDS Foundation. I recognized only a handful of veteran volunteers who had toiled with me earlier in the epidemic before we ourselves were swept away in the deluge. I did not recognize many of the Foundation's current clients. Those I had befriended at Foundation events in earlier years had all died.

The attending clients reflected a new population being ravaged. A few haggard gay men propped themselves up at tables populated now mostly with whole African-American families, a mother, a father both faltering; with Hispanic men, their tattoos draping on loose biceps; with street people bewildered at sitting in a warm room with people they dunned quarters from on the K Street Mall, some of them mumbling to themselves.

I found a place at a table among other gay men I did not know. I sat next to a sallow man in a wheelchair. I offered to get a plate of food for him at the buffet.

"Don't you recognize me?" he asked.

I looked more closely. "I'm sorry," I said.

He looked away. "Then I've disappeared. But, for the tombstone, I'm Jake Runyon. Or I used to be. You and I trained as volunteers together at the AIDS Foundation way back when."

"Oh, Jake!" I said. "It's been such a long time! Of course I remember you. You shook me awake when I dozed during the guided imagery exercises. And then I didn't see you around anymore."

"I moved to San Francisco soon after that training, hot on the slick, rose-scented trail of true love. That's all a hoax, by the way. I came back to Sacramento a couple of months ago. It's easier now living here in the Valley of the Dolls."

"How are you doing?" I asked.

"I'm trapped in hell's vestibule. As you can see," he said. "I can't walk. I'm fast going blind. I'm booked on the Coocoo Express and it's hurtling me to Dementiaville, the next stop. When I gather up my petticoats, toss my curls, and step down onto that platform, poof! I become a woman of mystery. Nobody'll recognize her. Hell, I won't either."

He started to sob. People around us paused in their eating, forks suspended.

I wish I were a person whose body glided effortlessly to enfold other bodies in distress, whose arms attended intuitively to comfort. I sat speechless. Jake's hands flattened against his face. Then he raked his cheeks upwards with the palms of both hands. "Hoo boy!" he said, and cleared his throat.

"I remember two things about you at that training," Jake said, his voice as steady as if there had been no outburst.

"That training changed my life," I said.

"Darling, you did not have a life before then," he said, patting my cheek. "I can still see you in those little plaid polyester Kansas button-down shirts from Sears you wore hitched up past your Adam's apple. You assured me everyone was wearing them on the plains. Anyway, to resume: I remember having lunch outside together on the second day of training. The courtyard was thick in trees with these brown fringy catkins falling all around us. Tiny orange birds darted about in the trees, jabbering. They were so magical. You were afraid they would shit on our heads."

"We had just had a lecture on toxoplasmosis," I said. "Birds were implicated."

"Toxo, yes. That's one ugly bastard that's glared at me across a crowded room but, so far, has kept his distance. His friends have all gay-bashed me, though."

"What's the second thing about training you remember?" I asked.

Someone set a plate heaped with turkey and dressing and peas in front of him. Everything on the plate blended the same beige. I remembered your Thanksgiving hospital tray of the year before. Jake looked the food over noncommittally and turned to me again.

"Remember that exercise we did on the first night?" he began. "We had gathered somewhere out on Greenback Lane at that ghoulish half-lit cemetery chapel so far away from midtown I thought I'd need shots and a passport? We had to write out the ten most important things to us on those ten cards we were given. Then someone read this thing about how AIDS robs people of all that is most precious to them, taking and taking and taking until there's nothing left. True story, by the way, though understated. At certain points we had to throw away two of our cards? Then later two more. Then two more. When it came to the last two, you wouldn't throw yours away. You tried to hide them or sit on them or something. You pitched a perfect little hissy fit, which left me breathless with admiration. They had to take the cards away from you, as I remember. What was on those cards?"

"I remember the exercise," I said, "but I don't recall what I had written on the cards." I remembered. On the cards I could not give up were my eyesight and my mind.

"Oh well, another mystery I must take with me to the grave, which is yawning for me right about over there." He pointed with a forefinger. "But let us try to eat. We need to keep up our strength. Oh yes, and our positive attitude, blah, blah, blah."

"What can I get you to drink?" I asked.

"Strychnine. Up. Very dry. Barbiturates on the side."

"I saw a pitcher of fruit punch over there. Will that do?"

"Yeah. A fruit punch. Just throw it hard enough to knock my brains out."

VII

I left about 3:00. The afternoon blew sunny and brittle. In the back seat of my car was a bright red present I would leave at your house for Joe. At the foot of the front passenger seat rested a miniature red rose bush in a terracotta pot for you.

I drove through the iron gates of Calvary Cemetery at 3:35. Tanners do not believe in visiting graves: your marker and those of your parents were bare as every day. I nudged the terracotta pot into the vase hole below your name plate. I thought of you lying deep in your concrete vault, clutching the ruby rosary in a darkness and a cold unbearable, the white blanket marbled in mold.

No one was out on your street when I drove up, the houses blind as if everyone had abandoned them and flown off in the Rapture. My key unlatched the front door to a cigarette-stale air colder than outside. Bonnie had left several days before to spend Christmas in Seattle. The rooms brooded in a dingy late-afternoon light. I had not been in the house alone since you were taken from it in late June.

Your bed was made up with the linens you had bought at Macy's almost a year before. I straightened the spread and plumped the pillows. Then I sat down. Bare Japanese maple boughs outside etched themselves onto the blinds drawn over the glass door to the garden.

I closed my eyes. Then began a crumpling. I found myself in a heap on the bed you had died in. What had been silent and beyond words for so many months now forced itself through. Finally. I do not know how long this lasted, this heaving buckle into snot and salt and spit. When after a time I could open my eyes, I saw myself in a mirror over the dresser. My face was a smear. I sat shivering in that cold house where I had been happy for a time.

At home, I cranked the furnace up high and turned on all the lights in the house. I began to pack for my Christmas trip to my family in Louisiana. I got the shoes out that I wanted to take. Next I put socks in piles, then trousers. A suit in a plastic cleaner bag. One of your ties. Then I arranged the suitcase, picking up piles from the bed and placing them for ease of access. I planned the carry-on—toiletries, a water bottle, the Sunday papers I had not yet read, what I needed for the flight.

I projected the next ten days in Louisiana and pieced them together, planned and mapped them, and I saw in that process the indefinitely protracted life task that now lay before me.

SEANCES

In the early months of your absence, I occasionally allowed my heart a dangerous license. Reason protested in loud alarm. I imagined you were still alive.

While standing at my sink washing a salad, I would make myself know you were sitting at the end of my dining table, your usual place, reading the newspaper in that focused way you had, waiting for dinner. You would not answer when I spoke to you. You checked the maneuvers of a faltering company in the business pages.

"Dore!" I would scold. "Are you listening to me?"

Or, I would call out from the bathroom while I was shaving to wake you for work, seeing you drowsing in white sheets while I glided the silver razor over my cheeks.

Or, walking in the fall woods by the river behind my house, I would call you to witness a merlot stain on an orange liquid amber leaf curling on the path.

I found it easiest to sense you in the front seat of my car while I drove to the Bay Area. I forced myself to think that a glance would catch you in profile, scanning the world rushing towards you through the windshield.

I do not believe in ghosts. I would not have you a glimmer down the hall, a chill gray smudge in a corner of a room. This was all a pathetic momentary palliative. Though my heart declared itself clairvoyant and demanded to be taken seriously as a medium, I always saw it tripping wires and throwing levers. It was all a cheap fraud.

My head demanded that I halt these vulgar reanimations, hold no more bogus séances. But my head and my heart rarely concur. My heart proved perverse in seeking you. It just could not believe that you could be gone for good.

One night a few months after you died, even my body, lumbering and dumb, fumbling for food and drink and dalliances in bed, woke to this matter. My body took the initiative here. Neither head nor heart was in on this caper. I stumbled home exhausted from a long teaching Thursday, including a night class. I drank a few glasses of a ferocious zinfandel and fell into a dreamless sleep on the couch while listening to the news on television. I woke with a start—loud laughter on some idiot after-hours talk show with Hollywood has-beens. I jumped up from the couch to turn the television off, afraid it would wake you. I tiptoed all the way downstairs before it came to me that you were not sleeping in the bedroom toward the back of the house.

"Do you think I need help? Maybe a therapist?" I asked Bonnie the next day. "I had to sit on the side of the bed for a few moments when I realized that I didn't need to tiptoe."

"You've tried the therapy route," Bonnie replied, "and it was a bust." She lifted her eyes to me: "We both miss him, Lu. But you're going to have to let him go."

TRACES

One morning Bonnie happened upon a shoebox heaped with photographs shoved into a far corner of your coat closet. It included dog-eared school shots of you, your face open and blank, the borders of the pictures scalloped. Bonnie held up a small black-and-white photo of you sitting on a rectangle of gray grass, a toddler, white as a milkweed float.

Other photographs edged you at the border of groups, accidental images: trudging up a ship gangway in a queue; lolling out of center in an airport waiting area; sitting in profile to the side of an office cafeteria table. Clearly these photographs you had culled as of little moment: pictures of you on the margin of other lives or on the periphery of your own.

I asked for the box. Two photographs arrested me. I propped them at the edge of my desk and gazed at them off and on for days.

In the first of these photographs, you sit in your square-cut bathing suit on the edge of a pool. You look up, squinting. Your legs look as if they have been broken off and re-attached at an odd angle below the water.

You are not the subject of this photograph. You sit on the side of the pool watching two young men grapple with each other on the shoulders of two sturdier men. You are on an all-gay cruise: men galore.

You are not alone. Next to you sits a man with shiny dark hair. He extends his arm out before him as if foreshortened in a Mannerist painting, twisting it as if to look at his elbow. He is lean and supple, tensed sexy. Dark hair feathers the dip in his chest between two dark nipples.

"He looks a little like you," Bonnie says. But he is not me.

Bonnie tells me stories I do not want to hear, traces of your life before I knew you. "He almost got 86'd from a gay cruise ship once," she begins. "During a night sail, he was discovered having sex on deck. They both had roommates who were tricking in their cabins at the time, so the two of them crawled under the canvas of a suspended lifeboat and went at it. Its swaying gave them away. Major safety breach, apparently."

Or Bonnie would go on about the Gay Games in New York, how on the first day there, she stood on a hotel balcony three floors up and watched you walk off with some guy you chatted with at the pool for maybe twenty minutes, both of you snatching white towels from your chaises, you coming back to the room two hours later to clean up and go out to dinner. No details offered.

"They all looked like you," Bonnie said: "Smaller, darker than Dore, preppy, thin, good teeth." But they were not me.

I have finished looking at the second photograph as well. You are the apex of a triangle anchored on the base by a couple, a man and a woman I do not know. They hold hands seated at a table, their ring fingers gold-banded. She wears a ridiculous white blouse with way too many pleats and ruffles. The man across from her smiles with his whole face: he is lithe and dark with a moustache stretched in a straight line. He looks a little like me, but handsomer.

At first you seem exactly centered behind them, but on closer inspection, you lean towards the man. Your hand rests on the man's chair back. The woman has pulled the man's hand over to her. You look out at the camera over their hand-holding with your frank eyes and diffident smile and hair-swept forehead, handsome as a Kennedy. An empty wine glass rises from the table directly before you: it aligns precisely with your dark tie. It is your emblematic portion in this picture: an empty vessel of clear, brittle glass.

My eyes roam the photograph. I am going to have this my way for once. Where the woman sits I force an erasure. I position you in her vacant chair. The hand you clasp is now mine. The man's features, already a little like mine, I trace over and reconfigure. I see myself in profile now, looking over at you. The man's smile I appropriate as my own. You have pulled your chair closer to mine.

The wine glass before us is now filled, its lucent bowl brimming purple.

HOW DO I LOVE THEE?

I arrived in Calaveras Hall five minutes before my 1:30 survey class in Victorian literature was to commence. We would spend this class on Elizabeth Barrett Browning's *Sonnets from the Portuguese*, a sequence of forty-four poems written in her astonishment at having fallen in love with the then unknown poet, Robert Browning, when she was a dedicated spinster of nearly forty years. The shock of that love ejected her from dim, cloistered London rooms on Wimpole Street, where she had lived as an invalid, into the oleander sunlight of an airy apartment on the *piano nobile* of the Casa Guidi in Florence. She writes of the violent miracle of her love as no less than a wresting into a new life.

I have always appreciated this sonnet-sequence for its language and imagery, though I have read the work condescendingly as sentimental. I have faulted Barrett for lacking the sinewy line and durable thinking of her husband's verse. I always imagined her readers to be little old ladies of both sexes sipping pale tea and discussing the autobiographical references in Barrett's sonnets at Browning Society meetings in basements of shingled Anglican churches.

I intended to teach the work differently this time around.

Three young women enter and take seats close together by the windows. All three are working gum. All three wear low-rise jeans and tight tees, baring midriffs that bulge way out over wide belts. Muffin-tops. No woman over thirteen without a personal trainer, perhaps a little bulimia thrown in on the side, ever looks good in this cruel get-up—but I am an aging gay man, so what do I know?

Gus follows them in, a handsome young man who has messed himself up bad with barrels the circumference of quarters in both ears. A good plastic surgeon should be able to stitch these gaps up when he repents. I lose hope, though, on reviewing the brocaded sleeve of colored tattoos covering his left arm. Body Graffitti. Gus sits, opens his book, and begins, I suspect, to read the sonnets for the first time.

Deborah force-marches a black book bag on wheels through the rows of desks. In her forties, she has the harsh, been-there look of having known hard knocks from a bad husband. She sustains herself every Sunday morning at the Vineyard Fellowship in Rancho Cordova, an antidote she has encouraged me to try, worrying that my fag soul repulses her stern God. We are currently at détente on that issue.

Steve enters, a former student of mine who had been teaching high-school English for ten years before having to give up his career for the health reasons etched in heavy furrows along his rubbery mouth, the sunken cheeks as if he were sucking them in, the hectic coloring, that dark haunting in the eyes. He told me at the beginning of term that his drugs have failed, that his doctors have given up hope though they still feint-box at HIV with new drugs that only drain him further. He keeps up the pretense with them. Meanwhile, he attends my class for the pleasure he derives from the works and from being in school again but without having to write papers or study for tests. He will be dead within the year.

Next to the door, always at the periphery of my vision, sits my friend Joan, who attends my courses whenever I offer them. She is a willowy blonde of ethereal perceptions, a blend of meditation and yoga and Rumi and Eastern mysticism and kombucha tea and new-age thought.

A young couple in love wheel their mountain bikes in. Tanned-over-pink and obscenely robust, Rich and Amy relate to each other matter-of-factly. Brenda follows them in, disgruntled at earning C's on all her assignments. She does not dispute my assessment of her work: she thinks, however, that I should take into account her learning disabilities. In her view, I am stingy in barring her from that shining land where all serious effort earns at least a B minus, no matter how flawed the academic performance.

Other students meld into the class core. They say little, write careful notes.

"General reactions to Barrett's sonnets?" I ask after calling the roll.

Deborah retrieves a blond streak from a crease at the corner of her mouth and says: "I hate how Elizabeth all the time debases herself. She's constantly putting herself down and propping her boyfriend up. I know that's the way it was back then, but for me it's humiliating."

"Why don't you locate some specific passages that show this while I get other reactions from the class." "Easy," she says. "There's scads."

Gus raises his hand: "I found the sonnets very moving. Barrett's attitude to love is exalted and inspiring."

"Oh, she's so gushy and unrealistic," Deborah breaks in, flipping the pages of her book crisply. "She never admits that she just wants to jump his bones. She coats her lust in gooey frosting and won't even lick the spoon. It's all a crock. I swallowed the big one myself once upon a time and look where it landed me after sixteen years of a lousy marriage and three kids: a seat in this class and what I've been calling 'my new beginning.'"

"First thing," I say. "For convenience sake, we'll refer to the speaking voice in the sonnets as Barrett's own, though note that the title of the work suggests the distancing strategy that she has translated these sonnets from the Portuguese. There's also a private play in the title in that Browning used with her the endearment 'my Portuguese' because of her brunette coloring."

While voicing this caution, I think how much I would have agreed with Deborah before I met you: love as human illusion to mask animal lust; as fiction to ward off existential loneliness. Love as glue binding breeders just long enough to raise their children; then, if surviving beyond that, drying into friendship, often without sexual privileges. An exemption from these illusions is every gay man's gift, if he keeps his wits about him.

"I have to agree," hesitates Rich: "Barrett's sentiment seems excessive. Her hackneyed version of romantic love is conditioned by her era and by her gender." His girlfriend Amy regards him with raised eyebrows.

Deborah does not wait to be called on: "Look at sonnet 3," she says. "Barrett diminishes herself as 'A poor, tired, wandering singer, singing through/The dark, and leaning up a cypress tree.' She makes an over-boiled noodle of herself in contrast to Browning, whom she exalts as a 'chief musician' playing for queens. He just so happens to look carelessly down on her from that height. Oh, please!"

"Yeah," says Brenda over by the window.

"But turn to sonnet 5," says Gus. "Here she <u>seems</u> to abase herself by allying her life, her very self, with ashes and dust. But then the sonnet turns warning: 'the red wild sparks' among those ashes will, if Browning stirs them up, blow into a blaze that 'shall scorch and shred/The hair beneath' those 'laurels on thine head.' She's cautioning him as to the vehemence of the passion he has awakened."

"Has love ever struck you so forcefully that it has tilted your life?" I break in. "Look at the very first sonnet, the opening of the sequence: here Barrett asserts she has read Theocritus in the original Greek, an accomplishment reserved for men who matriculate at Oxford or Cambridge in her day. Thus she positions herself as a woman with an intellect to be reckoned with, one not easily overcome by mere school-girl crushes or empty emotion. She presents love as onslaught. In spite of her formidable intellect, love comes over her so forcefully and without warning that she likens love to an intruder pulling her 'backward by the hair' and binding her in a 'mastery' against which she struggles. She thinks at first that this love is, in fact, the death she has long expected in her invalid chambers. Only later does she realize love's way with her. Can love indeed be so powerful? So overwhelming? Has it ever slammed into your lives, yanked you away from the life you've lived before it struck?"

"Gah, I hope it never does!" says one of the gum-chewers by the window. "Barrett here sees love as some pathological rape fantasy."

"Yeah," says Brenda. I make a note of Brenda's C-minus contributions to the discussion.

"How many of you agree with her?" I ask.

A majority of the class raises hands.

"Cynical so early?" I sigh. I am, of course, a hypocrite, I who dismissed love as a chimera for most of my life.

"I'll put myself on the line, then," I say. "I believe in prudence and caution in love matters, but I also allow that love can prompt the sudden transformation Barrett marvels at in sonnet 7 where she describes being 'Caught up into love, and taught the whole/Of life in a new rhythm.' In that new life, she feels unsettled and peers around anxiously in unfamiliar territory. She starts sonnet 7 with the realization that 'The face of all the world is changed' since first loving. For love, she gives up home, family, country, even her reputation as the foremost woman poet of her age."

"Maybe," snaps Deborah, "but it's still the same old female self-battering: He's great; I'm a trinket. He's brilliant; I'm dimmer than his shadow. He's master; I'll get his coffee. Did Browning write any love poems like these to her?"

"So far, I'm major attorney for the defense," I say. "I need help."

"Okay," says Steve, rousing himself to the rescue. "Note that sonnet 10 counters that all love—certainly including her own—is 'beautiful indeed' and 'worthy of acceptation.' Barrett realizes that 'love is fire' and fire burns with 'an equal light,' whether it consume fine flax or rank weeds. Barrett accustoms herself to love at last, at least to the point that she can say 'I love thee." In those new words, she understands herself 'transfigured, glorified aright,/With conscience of the new rays that proceed/Out of my face toward thine.' Love, she claims, can effect this transformation in the loveless and unloved."

"'There's nothing low in love, when love the lowest,'" reads Amy, glancing from her text to her boyfriend.

"This is the sequence's turning point," Gus ventures.

"One of them," I suggest. "Perhaps we might see this sonnet sequence as a vacillating evolution with forward advances followed by doubts and regressions. The speaker in the sonnets works circuitously forward from being mastered by love and overwhelmed by her lover to achieving a new mastery over herself and a provisional control over a foreign land she finds herself lost in." I look around the room. Students are busy writing in their notebooks. I give them the works:

"Love ends Barrett's retreat from the world. She breathes a more bracing air than she has ever moved in before. She ascends into a sunlight more dazzling than has ever warmed her. Is it any wonder that her way is unsteady, her vision faltering? As in all sudden conversions, the resulting changes are hesitant and uncertain, progress vying with reversions."

Students busily write in their notebooks. This sounds testable.

"In sonnet 14, Barrett instructs her lover how to love <u>her</u>," says Joan oracularly from her aura by the door. "'Love me for love's sake,' she demands, 'that evermore/Thou may'st love on, through love's eternity.' She tells him not to love her for any of her attributes or characteristics which she might lose or that he may grow tired of."

"Exactly!" I say. "Excellent reading! Does anyone see this happening anywhere else?"

After a brief silence, Gus, fingering the barrel in his left ear, points to sonnet 16: "Notice," he says, "she claims that if he invites her to love, she 'will rise above abasement at the word.' In this sonnet, she both surrenders and triumphs."

"I'd like to look at sonnet 32," says Steve. "It's pivotal, I think. Barrett says that when Browning first took his 'oath to love me,' she looked for a quick reversal. After all, as she says, 'looking on myself, I seemed not one for such man's love!' There's the old self-abasement again. She calls herself an old, worn-out, tuneless viola that would spoil a good singer's song. But then she acknowledges that picked up by his 'master-hands,' the 'defaced' viola floats 'perfect strains.' Here she raises herself from any abasement: her love, his for her, tunes in her her highest music. She calls it 'perfect.' Her song is perfected by their love, a high self-estimate indeed."

"Nice reading," I say.

"Oh, bull!" roars Deborah. "This is nothing more than a rehashing of that old Sleeping Beauty-kissed-awake-by-a-prince story. I don't buy it. She was playing her old viola pretty well before Browning ever took it up."

"Have you ever been in love?" asks Gus.

Deborah cocks a look at him as if he were a spider just rappelled down from the ceiling.

"We don't have to discuss 'How Do I Love Thee,' do we?" asks Rich. "All we need to do is consult our recent Valentine cards."

"We do, though," I say. "It's a rich poem, though over-quoting has made it a cliché. It's a fearless declaration of the love that has emboldened her in her submission to it. Here she shows she has learned love and commits to it fully, in this world and in whatever world may come afterwards. Note this sonnet's placement late in the sequence."

"The work as a whole is a moving tribute to love," observes Steve quietly.

"I find it so," I say. "*Sonnets from the Portuguese* offers a courageous examination of the risks and hesitant new certainties of a woman loving for the first time, much to her surprise. Barrett rights—or writes—herself after love's assault has ripped her away from her former life."

The bell rings.

Joan sidles up. Her advances always seem as if she is stepping out onto ice she does not trust to hold her. She tells me how much she likes Barrett's sonnets: "Just because I haven't always succeeded in the love Barrett writes of in my own life does not invalidate it for me," she whispers. "We are the ones who make love. Or fail it."

This is my last class of the week. I walk down the hall to my office. We in the early 21st Century have left little room for love to bust open locked doors and light the dim rooms behind them. Or expand closets. We have made sentiment suspect. I am a believer now: less than a decade ago I was a master skeptic. My refrain then: "I have seen enough of the damage done by what people call love. Let me just have a lot of hot sex."

I pack my book satchel, thinking of sonnet 23 where Barrett wonders "If I lay here dead,/Wouldst thou miss any life in losing mine?" My answer to Barrett's question has been the route of my recent life. It has written these pages.

I leave campus and walk home alone along the river. Spring is tardy this year, though it approaches at last. The dying light glows a cold green under new cottonwood leaves, glassy as the folded wings of the crickets now tuning silvery in the frail grasses edging the path.

LESSON THE BEAST

I became a love-atheist early on, intimations that I was headed in that direction appearing in my adamant repudiation of marriage to my mother in fourth grade. It took me close to fifty years to learn to love, or even that I needed the lesson. Slow learner. It took you only a matter of months to teach me.

In my defense, I maintained a reasoned denial of the reality of romantic love or any need for it. I grounded this denial in my understanding of the animal nature of human beings. Love does not figure for animals. Why should it for humans, every bit as animal as apes?

At every opportunity, we humans deny our animal natures, a renunciation of our essential selves. Perhaps defecation is the most obvious example: all animals shit in the same way physically. Unlike animals which simply drop their scat and are done with it, we humans are provoked to euphemism, frantically distancing ourselves from the fact that every human being cradles in the center of the body an intestinal vat of malodorous excrement. Like cats. Like rats. Like cattle. Certainly I would never advocate dropping our scat in front yards as dogs do. The point is we share identical physiological processes with animals, among whom we number.

In decay and death we find the ultimate human attempt to evade our animal natures. We die. Animals die. Period. What is the difference? Only that, for better or worse, we are aware of death and of our impending ends, which leads us to manifold forms of denial. Heaven? Hell? Resurrection? Reincarnation? All palliatives for the brutal fact that we, like other animals, are ephemeral creatures whose existences probably do not project beyond our mortal bodies.

Now to the point: Sex. I have seen dogs copulate. And rabbits. Birds too. I have seen myself copulate in mirrors set up to enjoy the view. I have watched porn. Regardless of the various fuckers engaging in it, copulation looks pretty much the same for all, except humans often do it face to face and we usually evince a greater awareness of our partners. So I have long thought that "love" is nothing more than an evasive fiction masking animal sexuality, an attempt to deny the raw, naked lust of the beasts rooted deeply in an animal nature we are ill-advised to deny. Sexual taboos were foisted on us to vanquish the animal body and its impelling erotic force. For me, for most of my adult life, sex was carnally celebratory, but only when at its rawest, and that meant not tarted up with "love."

Add to this the universal, usually religiously motivated denial to homosexuals of the legitimacy regarding sex and love extended to heterosexuals. Our sexual expression, the very fact that gay people indulge in sex at all, has been ruthlessly condemned by most human societies, offering punishments ranging from imprisonment to stoning to hanging, punishments as severe as those inflicted on insects or snakes just for existing. Cast out from the rules and conventions, sexual mores and marriages legitimizing heterosexual erotic expression, is it any wonder that I, a gay man so denied, would in turn deny the reality of love as defined to exclude me?

I have, of course, long understood that humans, as distinct from animals, possess a radical self-consciousness, that we inhabit both a symbolic and a natural world. I know also that our self-consciousness has declared war against the realities of our physical bodies. For so long, I deplored the near-complete victory of self-consciousness over the body, the successful attempt of human culture, the symbolic world, to transcend nature and thereby deny our animality, our essential identity. I still deplore it. Hence my denial of the existence of "love," that fiction tamping down full animal sexual expression.

I admit it: Part of all this I got wrong, but a significant part. I did not attend sufficiently to the strength of my own emotional yearning, to my own desire for self-expansion beyond a constricting animal nature, given as that animal nature is entirely to the satisfaction of its physical appetites. For humans, pure animality is a self-restrictive prison. The desire for self-transcendence which I came so belatedly to recognize in myself cannot be met when one's sexual partners are exchangeable, dismissible objects. I am not sure how it happened, but I discovered in you that the sexual promiscuity I had so long enjoyed and championed involved a contraction of the self to the body alone, a denial of other aspects of my humanity, like intimacy, like other-directedness, like tenderness and affection that are important to human fullness.

Nearing fifty, I felt at last the emptiness, the isolation, the aloneness of the pure animal state, but only after I met you. Loving you made me realize that restriction to one's animal nature can become yet another dark closet unless we open its door to let others in. The key to that closet door is love. You inserted that key into my lock at last. In you—better late than never—I moved from alienating and anonymous carnal encounters to a fusion of lust with soul-involving intimacy. My tardy recognition of this has apparently occurred to others long before me. Concurrently, I came at last to understand that compassion for others, like the many around me suffering from AIDS, is love's twin.

So at fifty, I became wiser: Love exists. You were my proof. This is a conversion narrative in a dark time. Even though love has led so many gay men to early deaths, love as cruel irony, love still remains the heart's yearning to fill its chambers with something more than bestial blood, as important as the beast's carnal imperatives are. Love results from the heart's need to be more than an animal-pump coursing salt fluids through a lumbering flesh bag.

The images of our love that remain to me lap at the rim of memory, high water marks:

A green comet hovers in a brown twilight, the western horizon a buff mesa, your hand golden in the last light.

The weave of your dress shirt after work, the sift of your hair short of the collar, your bristling against the kiss at the nape of your neck, shrugging the tickling away.

Your dissolving in a blaze of plum petals, fired by a sun dilated at setting.

Purple, rose, pearl rooms in a rhododendron architecture.

Scraping your uneaten plates into the wastebasket beneath the sink, the shrill of knife against porcelain. Clots of bile in a kidney-shaped basin.

Shadows pool lavender in the flanks of the red dunes we clamber up in early desert light.

Murmurs in shadowy rooms, the thrusting, the sighing.

You sit on an examination table under fluorescent lights, knobby knees dangling, deep indentures bracketing a mouth grim with endurance, and there is nothing to be done.

In a Mendocino garden, a sprig of narcissus in your hand exhales the fragrance of early spring. A hummingbird, flashing silver, shoots past you into shadows weighted blue.

"Let me go": an insistence in a darkened bedroom, everything coming undone.

Our martinis Mercury silver in a high auburn room after the swirl of curtains falling on the last notes of *Turandot*.

Your hair, morning musky; your breath raw on waking; the smell of your early flesh like no other scent, a sullen sexual perfume.

This is the sum total of first love for me: this stream of memories gathering together into a full reservoir. With you, Love became for me as real, as ardent as the new faith affirmed by an adult convert just emerging from baptismal waters.

AUBADE

It is the time's discipline to think
of the death of all living, and yet live.
--Wendell Berry: "A Discipline"

I am lugging a basket of dirty clothes to the laundry room of my condo in Palm Springs. At 11:30 A.M., my outside wall thermometer already registers 103 degrees Fahrenheit. I am startled to see one of the feral cats that roam the complex lying still just off the sidewalk, not quite under the pink hibiscus hedge. Its hind legs sprawl, matted in dust; its front legs array demurely, paws tucked under. It lies in the damp, cooler sand at the base of a sprinkler head.

I am shocked by the cat. It holds its head up but absolutely still. As I pass, it opens its eyes, olive and lusterless against its black fur, but they do not focus. They drift to the center and seem to look inside. They hold, beholding nothing. A stillness invests the cat, a patience, a waiting.

As I murmur soft pity sounds at it, I think of you dying, of that Friday afternoon with you in your bedroom. Sometimes, when I tried to talk with you, your eyes did not shift to me. They stared out, slightly down, not focusing. I did not know if you were fully conscious. A gravity, a severe isolation enfolded you.

When I returned to the laundry room to put my clothes in the dryer, the cat was dead, its head angled sideways on the sand, its eyes thin green gleams through closed crescents, its mouth glinting tooth.

Everywhere in the world I have for so long found you repeated, echoed, reflected since you died. A distant hill I note each time I drive the Cajon Pass rolls the exact contour of your shoulder under a sheet as you slept on your side. A sun-baked grapefruit has fallen onto the concrete surround of the pool I am swimming laps in. I catch its pebbled skin, singed a brown-gold, every time I turn my head for a quick breath, and I think of your fungal toenails, thickened and ridged yellow-brown. At the Walgreen's, I uncap a roll-bar of deodorant and smell again the antiperspirant you applied in the steamy bathroom as I shaved.

One morning this past April, I walked to work just after Easter along the bike trail edging the American River. I traced the tiny lavender bells tipping the coils of crown-vetch on the levee. I looked up to see you directly in front of me, your long face, your shy smile—but your hair had darkened and your eyes had deepened too blue.

"Professor Agosta," said this apparition, "are you in your office anytime today other than your regular office hours? I have a class then."

As he sat across from me in my office, late afternoon sun mottling us in shadow through the camellia bushes outside the window, I saw that only the contours of his high cheekbones, maybe the set of his chin were yours, nothing else, and these only a vague suggestion.

The car braking at the light in the lane next to me sounds the same high-pitched protest your white LeBaron used to whine. The eucalyptus outside my back door has leaves the shape of the quarters in the little tin bucket you kept your gambling change in, the coins green-silver in the shadow of the bucket rim. And last night the crescent of the moon over the purple mountains here in the desert traced precisely the bend at the center of your right eyebrow.

What am I to do now in such a world? Sometimes—when, for example, I closed the door to my office immediately after encountering the student on the bike trail—I think I must not go on like this. Grief has become its own end. I am pathetic.

Years ago, you asked me for permission to die: "Let me go, okay?" Now let me go, Dore. Let me go, okay? But I know it is not you who holds me. It is I who have never let you go, never fulfilled the promise you forced from me that last day.

I was having dinner with Bonnie on her recent visit to me here in the desert. She mentioned that you had always liked Palm Springs. She said she missed you. I told her I was much better now. She looked at me closely, at my downcast eye, and decided to risk saying it: "Have you really joined the living, as I asked you to?"

After you died, you seemed irretrievably gone. I clung tight to a dead body in that last bed. I could not let you go for so long because I dreaded the emptiness you left me in. In that void, I could not locate the living. I made the void reverberate with you and lived alone in echoes. But now I recognize that I am at last moving out from that long occupation. Writing this book has helped to bring you outside of me again with all the many others remembered here.

Now the world is becoming again familiar. The joy and sadness I found in you have at last urged me back to human fullness after a long absence. Writing of time and memory and love, of the loss of you and of so many others to AIDS, has worked its healing without my realizing it. Writing has gradually worn away the cell of grief like water eroding a limestone prison wall, at first allowing small darts of sudden brilliance in, finally crumbling enough to allow one to push out into open air and light. I am there now.

I am holding my love for you in my hand. It is radiant as dawn light. For so long, I have been using it to scan for you in a dark vault. I will extend that love before me now to illuminate the living world and my forward way in it to the end. Perhaps at that end, in some late dusk to come, I may stumble around a dark turning. In my death, I will drop that light. But there you will be, aglow in greeting, foremost among all those lost with you.

I have written myself out now. The fragments I gather of our having loved in the Losing Time no longer paralyze me. In these fragments the world again coheres; significances solidify; things mean clearly, and they mean well. I can let you go, Dore, as you asked. I will join the living now, in love and at last.

AFTERWORD

Following a man downstairs to bed, I looked over a thinning spot in his graying hair and at lines channeling the nape of his neck like roads scored on a well-traveled map, the ravages of sun over time on the skin of a man my own age, nearing sixty now. I felt a sudden tenderness for this mortal man, like a thawing that spreads over a winter land. I had hoped, but had not expected, to know again that opening to another first felt when I knew I loved Dore, and, after ten years have passed, the way I feel about him still—though without that vital force of love for a living man.

Bud turned to me at the bottom of the stairs to ask if I had rolled the trash can out to the curb.

"I love you," I said. "And yes."

His eyes softened: "Now what is this you're saying to me?"

Bud had crossed into love-language weeks before. "I love you, you know," he had said one evening as I was getting out of his car after a dinner date. He gauged my body's stiffening.

"I'm glad," I said lamely, and he had driven on.

Bud tried again one evening as we sharpened our shovels after planting apricot trees in the rocky clay behind his new house in the Sierra foothill town of Grass Valley. The setting sun backlit him in the Technicolor of the vow scene from *Gone with the Wind*. I rasped the file over my shovel blade, pretending not to have heard.

Bud grew bolder. The next time he told me he loved me, I was lifting a martini at sunset. He looked at me steadily, past retreat.

"I'm not ready for this yet," I had said. "And I'm not sure you are either." Bud's partner of twenty-four years had died of HIV-related complications five years before. Bud himself was HIV-positive. One of the fortunate ones, he took a single Atripla pill a day to keep the virus from doing its terrible work. He had an undetectable viral load.

When we had met almost two years before at the Bolt, Sacramento's leather bar, he had choked up as he told me about losing Daryl. That night was his first venture into the gay scene in the years he had spent grieving alone, traumatized and isolated, on his 89-acre ranch in the middle of beautiful nowhere. He and Daryl had built Keystone Ranch in their retreat from haunted San Francisco. Nearly everyone they had known during their twenty-three year sojourn in the City had died of AIDS. They had hoped to lay these ghosts to rest in open land, big skies above high hills, an immersion in a Nature that neither grieves nor remembers. But Daryl had died soon after moving there.

"I am ready," Bud replied.

I got a call from our friend Daniel who had introduced us at the Bolt. Daniel: over six feet tall, stunning silver hair, studly but somehow cherubic too. Nellier than 60's Barbie. Hell, even nellier than Ken. He opens his mouth to speak and a beaded purse falls out, a chiffon scarf wafts aloft. "I have to ask you something," he begins. "Promise me you won't get ugly."

"Ask," I said, "but I'll bet you're going to be minding my business."

"How do you feel about Bud?"

"Did he put you up to this?"

"He never would. It's just that I don't want him to get hurt. I met him during the bad years. . . ."

"I don't intend to hurt him, Daniel."

"Well, that's just peachy," Daniel sighed, "though short on pertinent details. You know that Mother likes all her children to be happy."

Daniel is sixteen years younger than me.

"You could maybe tell him how you feel? I think you could do it in just three short words, darling."

The words came that evening on the stairs.

"Dore gave you the beginning and the end of a relationship," Bud said later that evening in bed. "You both got cheated out of the middle years. I want to give those to you."

Once love seeds itself, it roots quickly. It leafs out green. All well and good. But love—at least for 60-year-olds—is very much of this world too. It cannot cancel the practical concerns of men each with properties and assets. The business of loving at that age requires strategy.

There were options: We could remain as we were—two individuals with two incomes, two houses, two sets of IRAs—clearly my first choice but perhaps not the wisest for two aging men looking to retire soon. Bud, being self-employed, was paying nearly a third of his income for health insurance—costly for anyone HIV-positive. If added to my employer-paid lifetime policies, he would cut his premiums by over 80%.

"I just cannot do the marriage thing," I told Bud during a walk along the river. "I'm happy the courts have allowed same-sex marriage in California for those who want it, but it's just too breeder-straight for me. I love being a badass sexual outlaw. I don't believe gays should go in for hetero-assimilation. Why do we need to join the military and go die in these useless Republican wars? And why do we have to ape married breeders and their inevitable progressions to the divorce courts?"

"It doesn't have to be like that."

"Maybe not, but I have floated through adulthood with a buoyancy I never see in breeders trudging through Wal-Mart towing cranky children and dulled by boring jobs, skimpy budgets, and bulging spandex. I want to stay gay."

"Whatever," Bud sighed. "But partners with imagination and energy can shape a marriage that suits them. There are no molds for marriage. We don't have to ape the straights."

"Just can't do it," I said.

"Then a domestic partnership?"

"I just wish we didn't have to go all legal."

We consulted an attorney to write up a pre-partnership agreement. "Is this to be a domestic partnership or a 'marriage'?" The attorney uttered this as if he were sluicing sour phlegm, bracketing the word "marriage" with two dismissive fingers from each hand. Air quotes. I had noted the attorney's desk photographs in full Knights of Columbus regalia shaking hands with a cardinal. And the framed invitation for the first inauguration of George W. Bush.

"I can draw up an agreement that will work for either a domestic partnership or a 'marriage' [the two-fingered dismissal again]. You can decide later which option will work for you."

"That was like inviting a gay basher to a Pride parade," I said out in the parking lot. "Why in the world didn't we find ourselves a gay attorney?"

The document served our purposes and was frightfully expensive.

The night following our review of this document, we were watching television. The airwaves were saturated with spots promoting Proposition 8 which sought to amend the California Constitution to define marriage as valid only between a man and a woman, thereby undoing the right gays had secured in 2008 to marry in California. One ad showed kindergartners forced to attend the same-sex wedding of their lesbian teacher.

"Teachers can't just hijack kids from a classroom like this without parental consent," I sputtered. "This is a new low."

"Have you seen the spot where the little girl tells her mother she wants to be a prince when she grows up? Her mother tells her she must mean a <u>princess</u>? 'No,' the girl lisps, 'my teacher told me I can be either one I want.'"

Outraged, I could think of little else for the next several days. A legal exclusion from marriage implies that gay people are unworthy of a public declaration that our love makes us whole. It looked to me as if the current freedom for gays to marry in California would be rescinded come the November elections. We were being out-spent on Prop 8 and out-maneuvered in the air wars.

Bud sat at my dinner table after supper, reading the paper. I knelt on one knee. "Marry me!" I said, collapsing the paper he held before him.

He looked away from me out into the shadows of the living room: "Where's the diamond ring from Harry Winston's?"

We decided to elope, the two of us saying our vows before some anonymous clerk—over and done with in minutes on a Friday morning. Applying for our license at the county office, Bud wrote his name in the new gender-neutral blank for "Party A" and mine under "Party B." He still refers to himself as "Party A" and to me as "Party Bottom." Sometimes that is correct.....

"What about monogamy?" Bud asked that evening. "I know it's never been a high priority of yours. If you agree to it, as I hope you will, we can re-negotiate at any time. . . ."

"Marriage!" I spat. "Already cramping my style."

I lay beside Bud, awake way too early the next morning. "I'm entering a doorway, not a box," I tried to reassure myself as I glanced at his hair gleaming dull silver in the wan light.

"You're anxious, aren't you, Luc?" Bud murmured without turning over. (Luc: I had left off using Lu as I approached retirement. Bud had never known me as Lu, a name I gave myself after leaving Louisiana in 1970 and which I had never really liked. So I had simply added the "c" to form a name I DID Like: Luc. Simple enough…. And if not now, when?)

"I've gone over it again and again, and I think I can do it," I said.

"Luc: sometimes it's just best to let things fall into place as they will. But I know control freaks like you have difficulty with this."

I ignored the crack, true though it was: "It'll be a good political move. We'll swell the ranks of married gays in case Prop 8 passes. We'll be in a wedge class, enjoying a privilege denied to others like us. That can't stand for long. And I'm good and pissed off: The constitutional rights of a minority are best decided by the courts, never by the varying prejudices of the public."

"Okay, Thurgood Marshall: can't this wait until coffee—say about when the sun rises?" Then Bud rolled over: "By the way, they want an extra 50 bucks at the courthouse to pay witnesses for our vows, unless we bring witnesses of our own."

"Let's ask Daniel," I said, "if we can get him up for an 8:00 wedding on a Friday morning."

"What will you wear?" Daniel fretted. "Hell, what will I wear as tramp-of-honor?"

"Jeans will do."

"I'm bringing Jack. He'll have to stand in as flower girl, but without the pinafore. We'll explode a magnum of champagne before the wedding to help me through the dawn, which, needless to say, I have heard of but never actually witnessed."

"Join us for a nuptial breakfast at Il Forno's downtown after our visit to the courthouse," I told my friend Mary T.

"You two will wear coats and ties!" she shouted. "I'm bringing boutonnieres. I'm also bringing breakfast to your house—frittata and fruit, appropriately enough. Also a wedding cake. Set your table for six. Robert's getting a sub at school."

"It seems two other couples are eloping with us," I told Bud on hanging up.

A tattooed youth in sagging jeans and his bride-to-be with ratted-up hair and violent makeup sat smacking gum and smirking at the six of us as we waited on the courthouse steps for the doors to open. Straight people, no matter their age or social class, have still a power that often makes me ill-at-ease.

"Any rings?" quavered the clerk in the midst of an arthritic half-turn as she led us, hobbling, down a hallway.

"Double-ring," I ventured, meeting Bud's startled look with a gesture to the silver band on my right hand. We had bought matching rings from a street vender with missing fingers in Mazatlan during a cruise down the Mexican Riviera to console me on turning sixty.

The clerk led us into a narrow wedding chapel fronted by a spindly lattice arch topped with two ragged accordion wedding bells. Strands of dusty silver beads looped through the lattice like cobwebs, fat and dewy.

"Oh, Diva!" Daniel frowned at the clerk: "Don't you have another wedding chapel we can use? Somewhere pretty?"

As I repeated my vows, holding Bud's hand, I glimpsed our reflections in a mirror placed at the end of the room. I stood, not alone as I had so long been, but coupled now for as long as either of us lived.

-- Married!! So much for my long-standing vow, taken at the prescient age of nine! So my mother had been right all along!--

Everyone in the room sniffled. Bud's voice broke. Afterward, Daniel tottered the clerk backward with a bent-over embrace: "So beautiful!!" he sobbed, "though this wedding chapel NEEDS me!"

I had set the breakfast table at my house with white roses and baby's breath, little white swans freighted with silvered almonds. The breakfast proceeded jovially, helped along by bottles of Moet-Chandon.

After clearing the table, I hesitated on putting away the bedside photograph of Dore and me taken in the twilit desert so many years before. Bud came up behind me: "You don't have to do that."

On our way to Bud's new Sierra foothills home in Grass Valley, we stopped at a nursery to pick up four tagged olive trees I had bought for Bud as a wedding gift. We would plant them together that evening. "Symbols of amity and of longevity between us for the rest of our lives," I said as we stood back to admire their silvery leaves against a setting sun in the day's last dazzle.

That night in bed, spooning Bud from behind, I could not sleep. His body had loosened from its tight compression and his breath came in deep draughts. I looked over the hunch of his shoulder at the moon that silvered the black hills beyond the window. I lay there, embracing a living man and remembering a dead one. And gratitude welled up in me for my having been given the grace to learn, belatedly, the realities of love, its sweetness, its bitterness, its power, all its sorrows and deep satisfactions. And here was Dore's final lesson, his wedding gift to me: Love need never die, though lovers do and years pass. Love grows once planted. And it can bear fruit in time for another. AIDS has no final power over it.

ABOUT THE AUTHOR

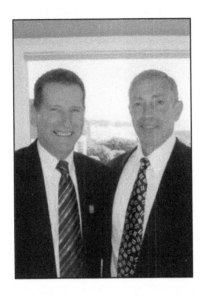

Lucien L. Agosta (left in photo), Emeritus Professor of English Literature at California State University, Sacramento, earned his Ph.D. at the University of Texas, Austin, in 1977. In addition to publishing numerous articles in his field, he is the author of two books: HOWARD PYLE (G. K. Hall, 1987) and E.B.WHITE: THE CHILDREN'S BOOKS (Simon and Schuster Macmillan, 1995). He appears on the DVD for the 2006 film version of CHARLOTTE'S WEB under the segment "What Makes a Classic." He is married to Bud Sydenstricker and now resides in Palm Springs, CA.